Young people's health — a challenge for society

Report of a WHO Study Group on
Young People and "Health for All
by the Year 2000"

World Health Organization
Technical Report Series
731

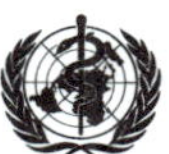

World Health Organization, Geneva   1986

ISBN 92 4 120731 0

© World Health Organization 1986

ISSN 0512-3054

PRINTED IN SWITZERLAND

85/6492 – Schüler SA – 9000

CONTENTS

Page

LIST OF TABLES

LIST OF FIGURES

STUDY GROUP ON YOUNG PEOPLE
AND "HEALTH FOR ALL BY THE YEAR 2000"

Geneva, 4–8 June 1984

*Members**

Mme M. Allain-Regnault, Société nationale de télévision Antenne 2, Paris, France

Dr N.O. Bwibo, Faculty of Medicine, University of Nairobi, Nairobi, Kenya

Dr E. Chigier, Youth Aliyah, The Jewish Agency for Israel, Tel Aviv, Israel

Dr P. Franzkowiak, Research Group Youth and Health, Heidelberg, Federal Republic of Germany (*Chairman*)

Professor O. Jeanneret, Institute of Social and Preventive Medicine, University of Geneva, Geneva, Switzerland

Dr R.O. Jegede, Department of Psychiatry, University College Hospital, Ibadan, Nigeria

Dr M. Knobel, Department of Adolescent Psychology, University of Campinas, São Paulo, Brazil

Dr S. Macintyre, Medical Research Council, Medical Sociology Unit, Aberdeen, Scotland

Dr U.S. Naidu, Tata Institute of Social Sciences, Bombay, India (*Vice-Chairman*)

Mr J. Paxman, The Pathfinder Fund, Boston, MA, USA

Dr M. Purificaçao Araújo, Consultant Obstetrician in Maternal Health and Family Planning, General Directorate of Health, Lisbon, Portugal

Dr E. Velásquez, Faculty of Medicine, University of Antioquia, Antioquia, Colombia

Representatives of other organizations

United Nations Fund for Population Activities

Dr J. Donayre, Deputy Chief, Policy and Evaluation Division, UNFPA, New York, USA

International Labour Organisation

Mlle M. Nussbaumer, Coordinator for the Question of Young and Older Workers, ILO, Geneva, Switzerland

International Children's Centre

Professor J. Guignard, Scientific Director, ICC, Paris, France

International Federation of Medical Students' Associations

Ms M. Klee, Danish Medical Students Organization, Copenhagen, Denmark

International Planned Parenthood Federation

Dr P. Senanayake, Medical Director, IPPF, London, England

World Association of Girl Guides and Girl Scouts

Ms I. Uygur, WAGGGS representative at the United Nations, Geneva, Switzerland

---

* Unable to attend: Dr Ye Gongshao, Research Institute of Child and Adolescent Health, Beijing Medical College, Beijing, China.

Secretariat

Dr M.A. Belsey, Chief, Maternal and Child Health, WHO, Geneva, Switzerland
(*Secretary*)

Dr D. Bennett, Adolescent Medical Unit, Royal Alexandra Hospital for Children,
Sydney, Australia (*Consultant*) (*Rapporteur*)

Dr N. Kapor-Stanulovic, Department of Psychology, University of Novi Sad,
Novi Sad, Yugoslavia (*Consultant*)

Dr A. Petros-Barvazian, Director, Division of Family Health, WHO, Geneva,
Switzerland

YOUNG PEOPLE'S HEALTH: A CHALLENGE FOR SOCIETY

Report of a WHO Study Group on Young People and "Health for All by the Year 2000"

1. INTRODUCTION

1.1 Opening remarks

A WHO Study Group on Young People and Health for All by the Year 2000 met in Geneva from 4 to 8 June 1984. The meeting was opened by Dr D. Tejada-de-Rivero, Assistant Director-General, on behalf of the Director-General. In his opening remarks, he emphasized how young people could contribute to, as well as benefit from, the WHO global strategy designed to achieve Health for All by the Year 2000. The aim was not the Utopian one of a world free from disease; what was sought was a society where there would be less inequity in health care and where health and wellbeing would be promoted through the active cooperation of all sectors of the community. Essential to the strategy was the strengthening of primary health care, a crucial factor being the active participation of the young people who formed such a large proportion of the world's population, especially in developing countries. While requiring the social support of the family and the community and technical support from the health sector, young people could play a part themselves in the choice and use of appropriate technology for the achievement of the desired goals.

The year 1985 had been designated as International Youth Year, whose theme was "Peace, Participation, Development". It was fitting that the Study Group should be devoted to harnessing the energies and idealism of young people so that the problems they faced could be tackled in a creative way. It was to everyone's advantage to provide them with trust and support by giving them responsibility and a share in the control of the technology and institutions affecting their future and the development of their communities. The Study Group had as its overall objective an examination of the health issues faced by young people and the broad social dimensions of those issues in a rapidly changing world, together with an exploration of ways of meeting the challenges posed by the active involvement of youth in the promotion of health for all.

1.2 Objectives

The specific objectives of the Study Group were as follows:

(1) to review the health and health-related problems of adolescence and youth (as defined below) in the context of current and emerging socioeconomic circumstances;

(2) to provide an analysis of existing health systems as they apply to young people in the context of primary health care, concentrating on their relevance, the availability of resources, and the gaps;

(3) to recommend strategies for the active involvement of young people in primary health care;

(4) to consider policy recommendations with regard to the health of young people and to suggest guidelines and priorities.

1.3 Basic considerations

Two major transitions involving young people are considered in this report:

(a) the transition of the individual from childhood to adulthood;

(b) the transition of certain societies from a traditional to a contemporary culture.

Both types of transition present challenges which young people are obliged to meet. It is necessary for both individuals and the social milieu in which they live to adapt to these transitions if health is to be achieved. Society must enlist the necessary support to enable individuals to cope successfully with the stresses involved and must foster adequate policies, programmes, and services to meet the special needs of young people.

The Study Group took a developmental view of adolescence as a period during which biological, psychological, and social maturation takes place. Youth was regarded as the period of transition from adolescence to adulthood. The Group urged that the views of the young be listened to and that their health and health-related problems be seen as rooted in the social, economic, and political realities of the world in which they live. It emphasized that the young people of today are capable of assuming responsibility for,

10

and are ready for active participation in, their own health care. Two aspects of health care were considered in this connection: the prevention of illness and injury, and the provision of services to deal with problems that have already arisen.

While this report cannot be considered as definitive, it is hoped that its broad scope will stimulate the exploration of a wide variety of ways in which young people may be used as a resource for the promotion of health.

1.4 Age ranges of adolescence and youth

Adolescence is the period of transition from childhood to adulthood, and it is characterized (*a*) by efforts to achieve goals related to the expectations of the mainstream culture and (*b*) by spurts of physical, mental, emotional, and social development.

While the onset of adolescence is usually associated with the commencement of puberty and the appearance of secondary sex characteristics, the end of adolescence is less clearly defined. It varies greatly from culture to culture as far as the attainment of adult independence is concerned. The transition is characterized by:

—biological development from the onset of puberty to full sexual and reproductive maturity;
—psychological development from the cognitive and emotional patterns of childhood to those of adulthood;
—emergence from the childhood state of total socioeconomic dependence to one of relative independence (*1*).

WHO had earlier considered 10–19 years as the period of adolescence, noting that this age range, which generally encompasses the time from the onset of puberty to the legal age of majority, coincides with some population statistics and is useful for health planning.[1] For the purposes of International Youth Year, the United Nations has defined "youth" as encompassing the age range 15–24 years. However, this commences in mid-adolescence, and its acceptance here would preclude a proper consideration of the special characteristics and needs of adolescents. A pragmatic approach to this issue is to merge the two age ranges into the all-encompassing range of 10–24 years, within which the three five-year subdivisions

---

[1] *Regional working group on health needs of adolescents: final report.* Manila, WHO Regional Office for the Western Pacific, 1980 (unpublished document ICP/MCH/005).

of 10–14, 15–19, and 20–24 years could be considered separately, where necessary. It is proposed that the term "young people" should refer, in general, to the composite age range of 10–24 years, although, in practice the terms "adolescents", "youth", and "young people" tend to be used interchangeably.

One advantage of such a grouping is that it facilitates cross-national comparisons of data and experience.

There can, of course, be no universally relevant categorization, and the proposed grouping involves a number of problems and constraints, including the following:

1. The subdivisions are necessarily arbitrary and, from the practical, clinical viewpoint, may involve conceptual constraints and contradictions.

2. The grouping does not acknowledge the discrepancies between chronological age and biological and psychosocial stages of development, nor the wide variations due to personal and environmental factors.

3. In both developing and developed countries, the concept of "young people" varies according to cultural and legislative factors such as compulsory age of schooling, accepted age of marriage, child labour legislation, and so on.

4. Age groups are of limited value where the precise ages of individuals are not known.

5. The development of programmes with excessively rigid age boundaries can be dangerous and there is a particular need for flexibility in this respect in the developing countries.

6. Other possible age groupings may be more useful in certain situations where local needs should have priority. For example, in the development of services and programmes for adolescents, the concept of early, middle, and late adolescence has relevance (see section 2.1.1). In the area of reproductive health and risks to health, the situation of young adolescents is markedly different from that of older ones. For some purposes, e.g., the analysis of morbidity data, information on a year-to-year basis may be more useful than any age grouping.

1.5 Demographic trends

Estimates suggest that approximately 30% of the world's population is currently between the ages of 10 and 24 years. Global population projections such as those depicted in Fig. 1 show marked differences between developing and developed countries.

Between 1960 and 1980, the world population of 15–24-year-olds increased by 66%, while the total population of the world increased by 46%. In developed countries the absolute size of the population of young people is decreasing, while in the developing countries it is rapidly increasing (Table 1). Of all 15–24-year-olds, the percentage living in developing countries was 77.6% in 1980, and it is predicted to be 83.5% by the year 2000.

One consequence of this huge increase in the number of young people in the developing world is the prospect of an even greater population expansion in the succeeding generations. Even if there were to be a rapid decline in age-specific fertility rates among young people, a stabilization of population growth would not occur for at least 10–20 years as the people in this "population bulge" reach reproductive age. Despite legislative attempts to raise the minimum age, the marriage of young women in their teens is still common in a number of countries and consequently a large percentage of the women in these countries have children before they are 20 years old. That this situation can be avoided is illustrated by the wide variations between countries in this respect (Table 2). Births to women under 20 years also represent an increasing proportion of all births, a fact partly explicable by the comparatively large number of young people in the populations of developing countries. Demographers have demonstrated that early child-bearing is associated with high total fertility.

As massive increases are also expected in the number of old people, resources will be further strained. Simultaneous increases in the number of adolescents and old people will produce competing claims for resources in the areas of health, income maintenance, and housing.

Perhaps more specifically in developing countries, adolescents will be particularly affected by the social consequences of demographic change.

1.5.1 *Mortality*

The mortality rates for young people are low compared with those for infants and the aged. Over recent decades, there have been significant changes in mortality patterns among adolescents, with a relative decline in deaths from infectious diseases and a relative

Fig. 1. World population by age and sex, 1980 and 2000 [a]

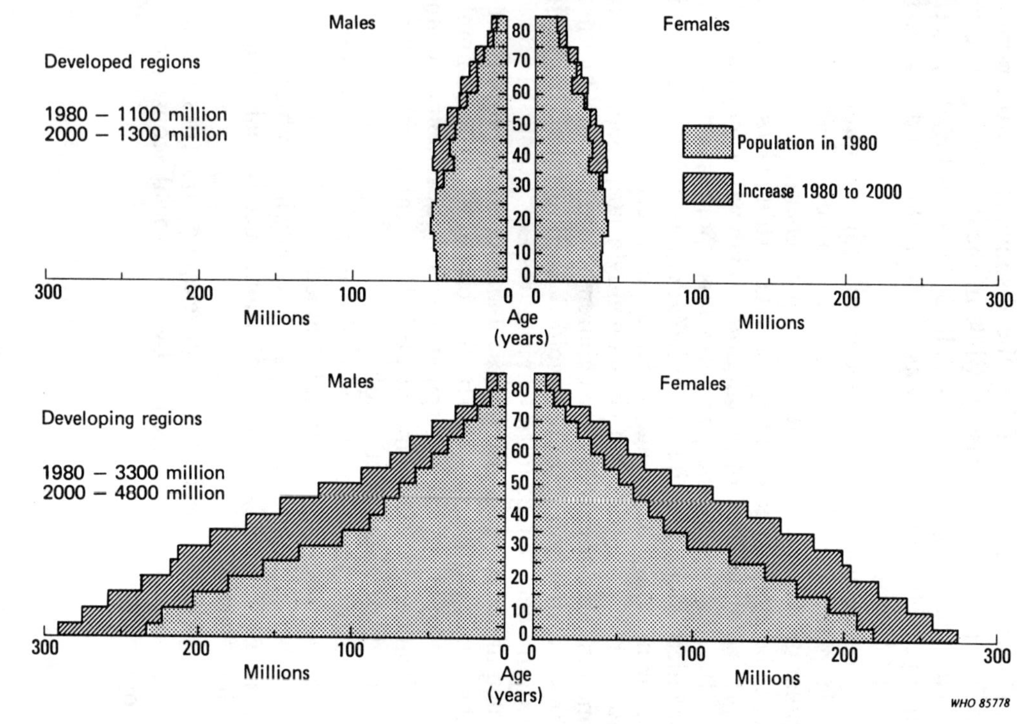

[a] United Nations estimates and projections as assessed in 1980.

Table 1. Population trends by age group and type of region, 1960–2000 [a]

		All ages		15–24 years	
	Year	Population (thousands)	Increase since 1960 (%)	Population (thousands)	Increase since 1960 (%)
Developed regions	1960	944 909		144 001	
	1980	1 131 339	19.7	199 512	38.5
	2000 [b]	1 272 159	25.7	176 253	22.4
Developing regions	1960	2 092 307		371 301	
	1980	3 300 809	57.8	664 696	79.0
	2000 [b]	4 846 690	131.6	892 857	140.5
World total	1960	3 037 215		515 302	
	1980	4 432 147	45.9	856 208	66.2
	2000 [b]	6 118 850	101.5	1 069 110	107.5

[a] Based on: WORLD HEALTH ORGANIZATION. *World health statistics annual, 1983.* Geneva, 1983, pp. 754–755 (Tables 21 and 22A).
[b] Projected.

Table 2. First births to women under the age of 20 years as a percentage of all first births (selected countries) [a]

Country or territory	Percentage	Year
Japan	2	1980
France	4	1980
Egypt	8	1978
Zimbabwe	9	1978
Mauritius	14	1980
Israel	16	1980
Jordan	18	1979
Malaysia	19	1979
Tunisia	25	1974
USA	29	1979
Uruguay	30	1977
Chile	32	1980
Costa Rica	45	1979
El Salvador	49	1980
Malawi	55	1977
Seychelles	55	1980

[a] Adapted from: UNITED NATIONS. *Demographic yearbook, 1981.* New York, 1983.

increase in accidental deaths. In developed countries, accidents, suicides, and other external causes now constitute the major causes of death in adolescence (Table 3). While the proportion varies from country to country, overall these causes are responsible for approximately half of all deaths.

Table 3. Accidents, suicides, and all other external
causes of death as a percentage of total deaths among
persons aged 10–24 years in certain countries
(latest available figures) [a]

WHO Region and country or territory	%
Africa	
Mauritius	47.2
Americas	
Canada	77.1
Chile	51.7
Costa Rica	52.4
Dominican Republic	21.0
El Salvador	49.8
Mexico	46.5
Panama	39.8
Paraguay	34.8
Puerto Rico	63.0
Trinidad	53.2
USA	76.2
Uruguay	50.2
Venezuela	60.7
Eastern Mediterranean	
Egypt	27.2
Israel [b]	52.4
Europe	
Austria	72.9
Bulgaria	52.2
Czechoslovakia	66.3
Denmark	68.3
Finland	66.0
France	67.1
Germany, Federal Republic of	69.3
Greece	57.1
Hungary	59.0
Italy	57.0
Netherlands	57.4
Norway	69.2
Spain	56.0
Sweden	66.3
Switzerland	74.7
United Kingdom	
England and Wales	57.3
Northern Ireland	70.6
Scotland	66.8
South-East Asia	
Thailand	38.4
Western Pacific	
Australia	76.5
Hong Kong	54.2
Japan	57.9
Singapore	47.4

[a] From information available to WHO.

[b] It was resolved by the Thirty-eighth World Health Assembly in May 1985 that Israel shall form part of the WHO European Region.

Pregnancy at an early age presents a particular danger for women and their offspring. Maternal and child mortality and morbidity in relation to pregnancy are higher in the age group 15–19 years (and younger) than in women in their twenties (see data for maternal mortality in Tables 15 and 16 on pp. 61–62).

2. DEVELOPMENT IN ADOLESCENCE AND YOUTH

2.1 General principles of development

Development in adolescence and youth follows the general principles underlying all human development. These principles can be briefly stated as follows:

1. Development involves the gradual replacement of simple by complex structures and functions.

2. Development is both continuous and intermittent. That is, some steps are dependent upon previous development, and some attributes and functions develop fairly independently of past experience and established structures.

3. Development is dependent upon an interaction between genetic and environmental factors.

2.1.1 *Adolescence*

Adolescence is a distinct phase of development. Its characteristics essentially depend on the ways in which biological, psychological, and social factors combine to fashion the maturational patterns involved. Despite individual differences and environmental factors, some of its features are common to all cultures. The developmental processes are characterized by periods of rapid change, interspersed with phases when there is an apparent loss of momentum with what, at times, appears to be a regression to earlier patterns of behaviour. Thus adolescents often irritate adults by acting childishly after seeming to have achieved acceptable standards of maturity. Development is often uneven. For example, the biologically influenced early maturation (i.e., the more mature appearance) of a young female adolescent may lead people to have social expectations of her that she is not yet ready to fulfil.

The average adolescent is faced with the resolution of a number of *developmental tasks,* including the following:

(*a*) adaptation to the physiological and anatomical changes associated with puberty and the integration of a mature sexuality into a personal model of behaviour;

(*b*) the progressive resolution of earlier forms of attachment to parents and family, and development through peer relationships of an enhanced capacity for interpersonal intimacy;

(*c*) the establishment of an individual identity incorporating a sexual identity and adaptive social roles;

(*d*) the utilization of enriched intellectual competence with the acquisition of a sense of community and a "world view";

(*e*) the development of potentials for occupational and leisure activities with a gradual commitment to those that are relevant to both the individual and the community.

The concept of developmental tasks is useful in a number of ways: it leads to a better understanding of patterns of progressive development in adolescence; it facilitates comparisons of individuals and groups of adolescents against developmental baselines; it provides a logical basis for understanding adolescent disorders, disabilities, and problems as being determined by, or shaped through, failures in developmental progress; and it can help adolescents not only to develop but to understand and respond better to explanations of their problems.

These tasks, of course, overlap to some extent, but the emphasis changes as adolescence progresses. In early adolescence, i.e., from about 10 to 14 years, attention is focused on developmental tasks (*a*) and (*b*). In middle adolescence, (14–17 years), the emphasis shifts to tasks (*b*), (*c*) and (*d*). By late adolescence, (17–20 years), tasks (*a*), (*b*), (*c*), and (*d*) are largely completed and the emphasis shifts to task (*e*).

This general sequence is, however, affected by socioeconomic and cultural conditions which may delay development through lack of opportunity. Indeed, the frustrations that arise in the absence of an outlet for the creative energy of the young may be at the heart of many of the problems associated with adolescence.

2.1.2 *Youth*

Youth, as defined by the Study Group, overlaps with middle and late adolescence; the concerns of the age group 20–24 years are, however, adult in their orientation. This group is characterized by increased stability and more outwardly directed tasks and activities, including:

(*a*) the formation of a firm capacity to make ongoing commitments in personal relationships, in the vocational sphere, and in other social contexts;

(*b*) a progressive assumption of greater responsibility in relation to parental figures;

(*c*) active commitment to working with established social structures.

Cultural factors influence the range and expression of the developmental tasks of adolescence and youth. In some cultures, these tasks are taken up, perhaps precociously, though by necessity, in early adolescence. Conversely, in other cultures, the opportunity to embrace those tasks may be delayed until middle adulthood. In either case, their major practical significance is the way in which they can focus attention on appropriate programme development. Where the opportunity exists, failure to exercise it may serve as an indicator of those young people at risk of, or already suffering from, disorders or disabilities.

2.2 Physical changes during adolescence

2.2.1 *Secular changes*

Over the past 100–150 years, there have been changes in the physical aspects of adolescence. The age of onset of sexual maturation has been decreasing, growth and physical development are proceeding at an accelerated pace, and there has been a trend (until recently) toward greater ultimate adult size. The age of menarche in Europe has become earlier by 2–3 months per decade, and there is a similar secular trend in the USA (apparently levelling off at about 12.8 years). Many aspects of this acceleration remain obscure, although such factors as better nutrition and improved social and economic conditions are probably relevant.

2.2.2 *Puberty: norms and variations*

Considerable changes in hormone secretion occur during adolescence (*2*), (Fig. 2 and Fig. 3). The first event in puberty is an increased secretion of gonadotrophic hormones by the pituitary

Fig. 2. Hormonal changes in relation to puberty in girls[a, b]

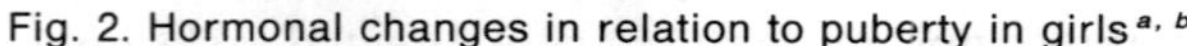

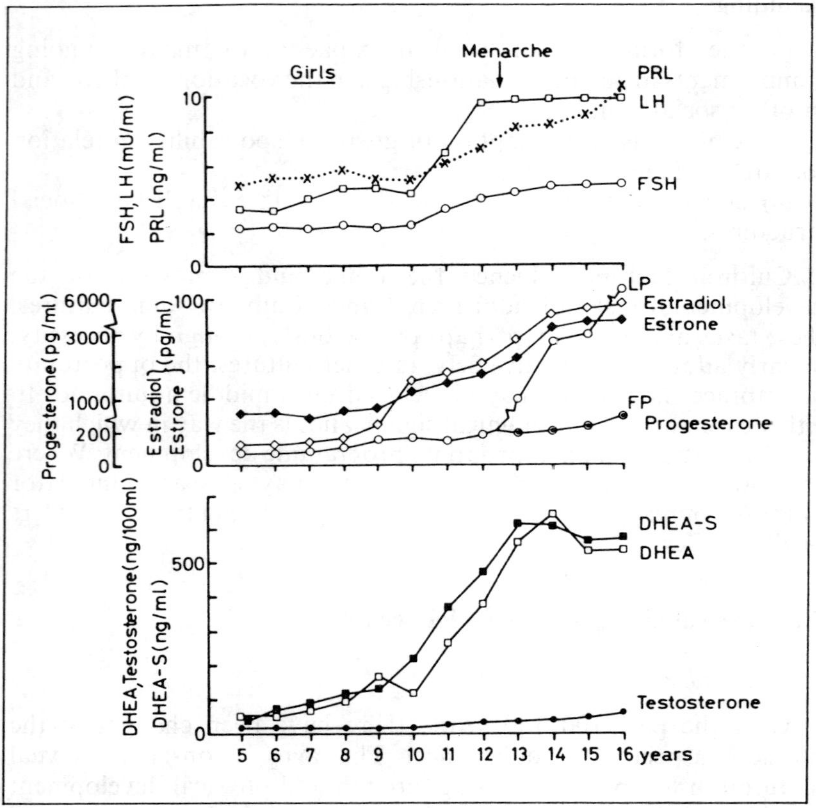

[a] Levels of plasma prolactin (PRL), luteinizing hormone (LH), follicle-stimulating hormone (FSH), estradiol, estrone, progesterone (before puberty and after menarche), dehydroepiandrosterone (DHEA), cehydroepiandrosterone sulfate (DHEA-S), and testosterone before, during, and after puberty in normal girls. LP and FP represent progesterone levels during the luteal phase (open circles) and follicular phase after menarche (dotted circles).

[b] Source: SIZONENKO, P.C. Endocrinology in preadolescents and adolescents. I. Hormonal changes during normal puberty. *American journal of diseases in childhood,* **132**: 704–712 (1978).

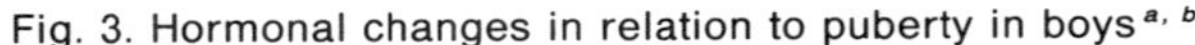

Fig. 3. Hormonal changes in relation to puberty in boys [a, b]

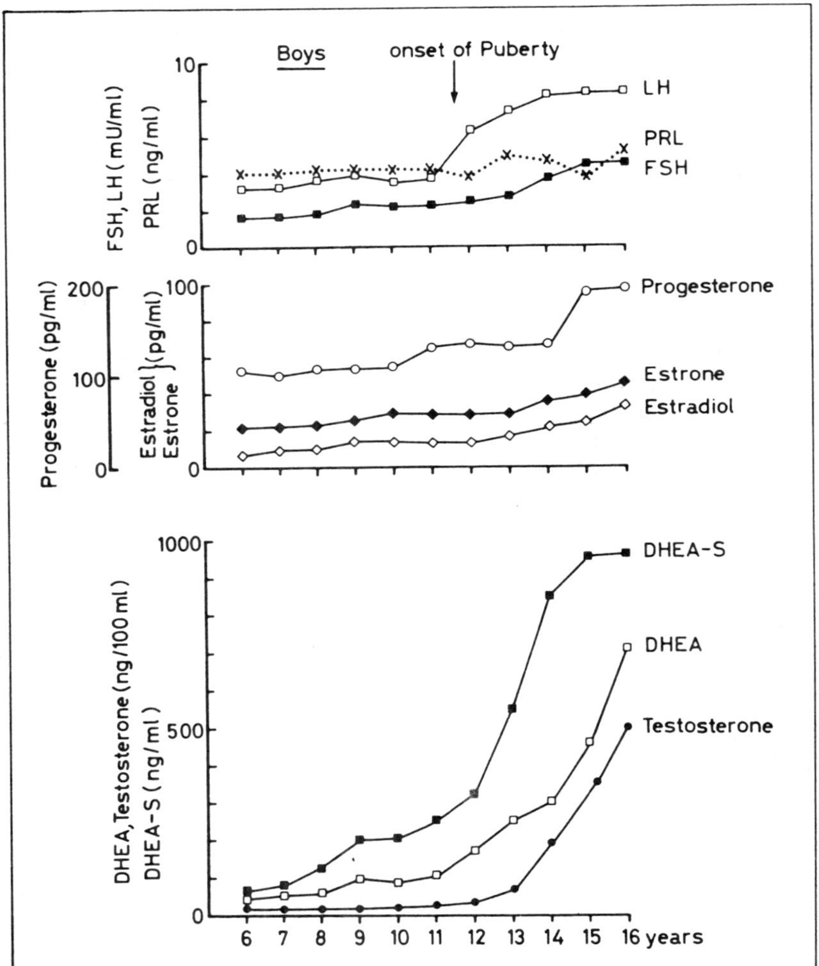

^aLevels of plasma prolactin (PRL), luteinizing hormone (LH), follicle-stimulating hormone (FSH), progesterone, estrone, estradiol, dehydroepiandrosterone (DHEA), dehydroepiandrosterone sulfate (DHEA-S), and testosterone before, during, and at end of puberty in normal boys.

^bSource: SIZONENKO, P.C. Endocrinology in preadolescents and adolescents. I. Hormonal changes during normal puberty. *American journal of diseases in childhood*, **132**: 704–712 (1978).

gland, which causes the follicles of the ovaries and the tubules of the testes to develop. Estrogen production remains low, but roughly constant, in both sexes up to the age of 7 years and then rises gradually. As puberty begins in girls, estrogen levels rise sharply and estrogen production becomes cyclic. In boys, estrogen production also increases slightly during puberty, but the main change is a very large rise in testosterone secretion. In both boys and girls, adrenal androgens, which are already being increasingly secreted during childhood (3), also increase greatly at puberty, and these are responsible for the emergence of some of the secondary sexual characteristics, particularly pubic and axillary hair (adrenarche).

The first sign of puberty in boys is usually an enlargement of the testes, probably associated with the onset of spermatogenesis before the acquisition of male secondary sex characteristics. The growth of pubic hair is followed by spurts in height and in penis growth. Axillary and facial hair appear, on average, some two years after the growth of pubic hair begins; the growth of body hair begins a little later and continues until well after puberty. Voice changes related to enlargement of the larynx occur relatively late in adolescence and can take 1–3 years to complete. There is a permanent increase in the size of the breast areola and sometimes temporary enlargement of the underlying breast tissue in boys, which may cause discomfort or embarrassment. "Spermarche", the first ejaculation, usually occurs during sleep or as a result of masturbation in the middle or final stages of puberty (4).

The average duration of puberty is about 3 years, but it can last from 2 to 5½ years in boys and from 18 months to 5 years in girls. While the visible events of puberty follow a predictable sequence, there are wide variations in the time of onset, the rate of change, and the age of completion of these events. Breast development in girls, beginning between 8 and 13 years, is usually the first sign of pubescence (thelarche). It is followed, within a year or so, by the appearance of pubic hair, a height spurt, and changes in general physique. Once again, however, there is considerable individual variation in the order and timing of these physical changes, both within and between cultures.

Menarche occurs quite late in puberty and is generally preceded by at least 2 years of breast development. The average age of menarche throughout the world is about 13 years, but the range extends from about 10 to 16½ years. Cross-sectional studies have indicated a slight delay in menarche in rural as compared to urban

Table 4. Median ages of menarche at seven study centres, and ages by which 10% and 90% of the girls surveyed at each centre had all reached menarche[a]

Centre	10th Percentile		Median		90th Percentile	
	Years	Months	Years	Months	Years	Months
Hong Kong	11	2	12	9	14	2
Zafed (Israel)	11	9	13	3	14	6
Ile-Ife (Nigeria)	12	3	13	9	15	0
Colombo (Sri Lanka)	12	1	13	6	15	0
Peradeniya (Sri Lanka)	13	1	14	5	—	—[b]
Stockholm (Sweden)	11	4	13	3	14	4
Geneva (Switzerland)	11	4	13	1	14	4

[a] Reproduced, by permission, from: WORLD HEALTH ORGANIZATION. A multicentre cross-sectional study of menarche. *Journal of adolescent health care* (in press).

[b] At the conclusion of this study fewer than 90% of the girls had reached menarche.

populations (Table 4). While the reasons for this are not fully understood, such factors as socioeconomic class, altitude, family size, and nutritional status may be relevant (5). Proposed longitudinal studies may elucidate this matter. One idea put forward was the "critical weight" hypothesis (6), which postulated that menarche is directly related to body weight and possibly triggered by feedback from the metabolic mass of the body to appropriate regulatory systems. Subsequent studies (7) have indicated that weight unrelated to age is not likely to be the primary trigger of menarche.

It is worthy of note that menarche and spermarche do not necessarily represent signs of fertility. Early menses are usually non-ovulatory, and sperm released at spermarche is probably of low fertility.

2.2.3 *The growth spurt*

Longitudinal studies of physical growth clearly show that adolescence is associated with marked changes in both the tempo and nature of growth and development. The rate of physical growth progressively decreases from the fourth month of fetal life onwards until there is a marked acceleration during adolescence—the so-called adolescent growth spurt. Testicular androgens and estrogens are of major importance, although adrenal androgens may also play a role, before and during puberty. In the United Kingdom, the typical girl begins the adolescent height spurt at about 10 ½ years and reaches the peak rate of height increase at approximately 12 years; the boy begins his spurt and reaches his peak approximately 2 year later, the boys' peak rate being greater than the girls'.

It is important to recognize that there is great individual variation in the age at which the growth spurt occurs. It is accompanied by marked changes in physique, the changes being different in the two sexes in a way not apparent before puberty (*2*). Girls have a particularly large growth in hip width, whereas boys increase most in shoulder breadth. Both sexes show an increase in muscle bulk, but this increase is much more marked in boys than girls. Boys also show a very marked increase in strength, whereas this is scarcely apparent in girls. The bones thicken and widen, and the dimensions and shape of the face alter—more so in males than females. The head, hands, and feet reach their adult size earliest, so that some adolescents complain of having large hands or feet. Boys on average lose fat at adolescence with a further gain as height growth slows down. Girls show a similar curve but there is only a temporary slowing (rather than a loss) in accumulation of limb fat, and a steady rise in body fat, together with a general tendency to lay down fat as they cease to gain height.

2.2.4 *Psychological impact of biological change*

Both the nature and the timing of the physical changes of adolescence seem to be of psychological significance and to affect behaviour. The role of sex hormones in relation to physical maturation is clear, but their effects on emotions and behaviour are less so. It is evident from a variety of studies (*8*) that androgens have an important (but far from exclusive) controlling function as regards sex drive in the male. They probably have a similar effect in the female, being secreted by the adrenal gland. Thus, the rise in androgen production at puberty is responsible for the accompanying marked increase in sex drive which is a such feature of adolescence. However, it does not follow that differences in hormone level account for individual differences in libido after puberty, and the evidence suggests that in fact the links are quite weak. Androgens play a major role in the initiation of the rise in sex drive in puberty, but thereafter variations in sex drive (either between individuals or within individuals over time) occur which are not primarily determined by hormone levels.

The emotional and behavioural consequences of the changes in estrogen and progesterone levels that occur in adolescence are less well understood. But, from the proven evidence of the effect of hormonal changes on behaviour in other areas (e.g., postpartum disturbances, premenstrual tension, etc.), it is likely that the hormonal changes characteristic of girls at puberty have emotional consequences.

The timing of physical maturation during adolescence also has psychological significance. A number of studies have shown that early maturing boys have a slight advantage in personality (9). In general, there is a tendency for them to be more popular, more relaxed, more good natured, and generally more poised. In contrast, late maturers tend to feel somewhat less adequate, less self-confident, and more anxious. However, the personality tests used in the studies in question were not very satisfactory, and the differences observed were usually quite small. The picture emerging from studies of girls has been less consistent: the differences between early and late maturers have been less marked and have varied according to age and in different studies, with early maturation sometimes an advantage and sometimes a disadvantage. The early maturing girl may sometimes experience self-consciousness and anxiety and attempt to conceal breast development through altered posture. On the other hand, sexual readiness may not be concomitant with the psychosocial maturity necessary for satisfactory relationships.

2.3 Psychological development

2.3.1 *Cognitive and value system development*

Piaget (*10*) has been most influential in postulating discrete stages of cognitive development, which always occur in the same order, although the time of onset varies from individual to individual. At about the age of 12 years, young people first become capable of "formal operations", that is, the ability to manipulate hypotheses or propositions in the absence of concrete or tangible referents—in other words, systematic and rational abstract thinking.

Piaget has also postulated significant differences between the young child's moral functioning as compared to that of the adolescent. He describes the gradual shift from acceptance of adult norms and rules to the stage of critical evaluation of these rules, in which an active individual choice is made. This, in turn, creates conflict between the adolescent and authority figures; however, the degree to which that occurs may vary considerably from culture to culture.

2.3.2 *Identity formation*

Identity can be considered as an inner sense of being and belonging within the limitations and possibilities of each period of life. During adolescence, its achievement demands a shift from childhood roles to those of youth and adult life.

Instead of talking about an "identity crisis", many authors prefer to accept that anxieties about the future increase during the teenage period. In contrast to the concept of adolescence as a time of identity confusion and uncertainty about the self, there is the observation that adolescents tend at times to have unrealistically high opinions of themselves, though this has not received full empirical support. Studies suggest that in most respects adolescents have a fairly realistic view of themselves, although this tends to change from day to day. As children pass through adolescence they become markedly more able to generate and explore hypotheses, to make deductions and to achieve higher order abstractions. Adolescents' questioning and criticism of established views and their idealism are probably as much a function of their greater cognitive capability as a response to their social situation or pattern of upbringing.

2.3.3 *Adolescent relationships with adults and peers*

In "western" societies, adolescence has often been seen as a period during which young people become alienated from their parents, the result being a "generation gap", while their peers have relatively more influence on them than their parents do. While it is true that adolescents tend to have intense emotional interactions with their peers and a great need for their approval, this does not necessarily mean that they turn away from their parents. In fact, the empirical evidence consistently contradicts the commonly accepted view that adolescents tend to diverge from their parents' values and that parental influence is greatly diminished during adolescence (*11*).

Fig. 4 shows this positive relationship in that the vast majority of 14- and 15-year-olds included in an English study, believed that their parents approved of their friends and that a significant number of them still went on family outings. Only small percentages showed signs of being significantly alienated.

26

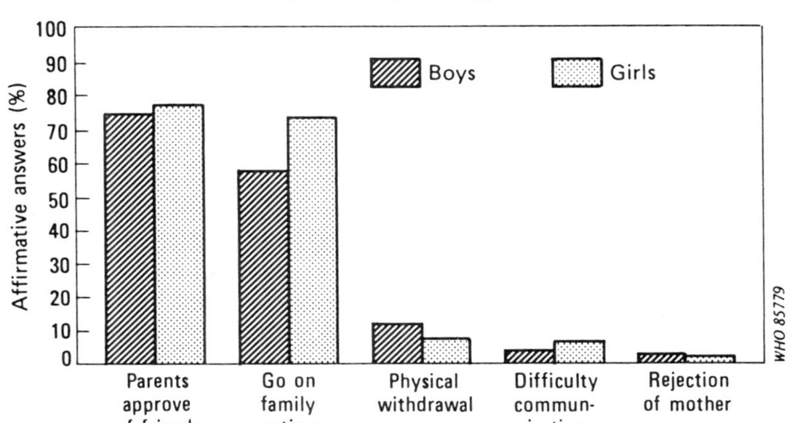

[a] Adapted from RUTTER, M. *Changing youth in a changing society*. London, Nuffield Provincial Hospitals Trust, 1979.

In general, the evidence seems to indicate that adolescents still tend to turn to their parents for guidance on major questions of values, but look more to their peers in matters concerning fashions in clothes, leisure activities, and other interests of youth.

2.3.4 *Societal factors in adolescent development*

In today's transitional societies, new stresses have arisen from the frequently wide divergences in experience and life-style between parents and their adolescent offspring. In the urban areas of developing countries, young people are facing problems and opportunities very different from those of their parents. Especially when the family is rural in origin, it is more difficult for them to turn to their parents for support and guidance. In rural areas as well, the spread of other values by the mass media is creating differences in attitude between generations. However, it should also be noted that the strengths inherent in traditional societies may be channelled in new directions, and account should be taken not only of young people with problems, but also of those who have adapted successfully and how they did so.

As noted above, both individual and societal factors affect the extent of development during adolescence and youth. While the sequence of developmental stages appears to have biological origins, the timing and extent of development are affected in varying degrees by environmental factors. Individual maturation in the physical, cognitive, emotional, social, and economic spheres rarely proceeds evenly and, in the best of circumstances, the completion of the developmental tasks characteristic of adolescence may be impeded by a lack of opportunity. Sometimes, there may be a loss of opportunity as a result of behaviour, for example, in the case of unprotected intercourse leading to an unwanted pregnancy, or that of drug or alcohol abuse, but such behaviour often has its origin in a lack of economic or educational opportunity in a society where increasingly complex demands are made on young people and traditional family support is weakened.

As technology grows more complex, more education and training are needed to achieve economic independence. As reproductive maturity is largely biological in origin, while economic independence is more often a result of national and international factors, the young person is often trapped between a growing sense of individual maturity and a lengthening of economic dependence. In traditional rural societies, the transition from childhood to adulthood is fairly short, with predetermined roles waiting to be assumed. In modern affluent societies, more support is available for young people over the longer periods of training and education required if they are to fit into technologically sophisticated economic systems. In the transitional societies that are perhaps most common in developing countries, economic necessity has weakened the authority of the traditional support system in rural areas and, at the same time, attracted young people to urban industrial areas where skills are at a premium, but support for training is in short supply. For a young person who is experiencing the natural stresses of the transition from childhood to adulthood anyway, the tension is heightened, the frustration compounded, and the likelihood of problems increased.

However, as pointed out above, it is important to consider the successful adaptors in transitional societies as well as those who have succumbed to problems. Each culture has unique characteristics which may facilitate adaptation in ways as yet unknown elsewhere. The very changes that are taking place may furnish new models for the participation of young people in social development.

3. SOCIAL FACTORS AND CHANGES AFFECTING YOUNG PEOPLE'S HEALTH

The preceding section was particularly concerned with the changes that occur in an individual as he or she develops from childhood to adulthood. In this section, we turn to the social factors that shape individual development, and to social changes that affect the development, status, and health of young people.

3.1 Cross-cultural variations in the concepts of "adolescence" and "youth"

While definitions of stages of development such as "adolescence" or "youth" in terms of chronological age are useful for purposes of standardization, it is important to recognize that they are socially arbitrary. A 15-year-old, for example, might well be considered a "youth" in one society, a mature adult in another, and a child in yet another. In the least developed societies, the age group 15–24 years is likely to constitute an important productive asset to the family and society, with others dependent on it, while, in the most developed societies, a large proportion of 15–24-year-olds are dependent on others.

Cross-cultural differences can also be seen in the variety of laws or customs on the minimum age for marriage, which is often different for men and women, implying differing views about the ages at which the sexes mature. Europe has the highest legal and actual marriage ages and is the only region where countries have the same legal minimum ages for both sexes. In some countries of Asia, the legal minimum age is low, and child marriage is common, though illegal, in Bangladesh and parts of India. Some Eastern Mediterranean and North African countries have no minimum legal age for marriage, choosing to adhere to Muslim laws which allow girls to marry at menarche. Others have moderately high legal ages, as do many African countries south of the Sahara. Latin America, on the whole, has the lowest legal ages in the world.

Several writers have emphasized that "adolescence" is a relatively recent concept and one mainly confined to modern "western" societies (*12*). In many different cultures there are rites of passage, in which the child (or, as some might say, the adolescent) is initiated into the social roles of adulthood. For males in such cultures, psychological and social maturity may only rarely converge. For females, ceremonial transitions such as betrothal or marriage may be closely linked to physical events such as first menstruation, but again not to full psychological maturation. In other societies, there are no such ritual changes in status, and childhood merges into adulthood without any discrete, intermediate status being perceived or labelled as anything equivalent to the idea of "adolescence". Modern ideas about this stage of life have been shaped by the introduction and extension of compulsory education, by laws prohibiting the employment of juveniles, and by the development of laws and services differentiating juveniles from adults or children. They have also been influenced by the increasing discrepancy between the age at which physical maturity is reached and the age at which economic, civil, and social independence is achieved or granted (*12*).

3.2 The importance of social factors

In common with people of all ages, young people find their life experiences shaped by the society in which they live. Their development, status, patterns of everyday life, aspirations, opportunities, and health are all affected by the nature of their society. Their lives are affected by legacies from the past: accumulated beliefs, laws, customs, and values (culture); the effects of earlier patterns of fertility, marriage, morbidity, and mortality (demographic patterns); the results of industrial, economic, agricultural, and political development (socioeconomic or sociopolitical patterns); and the consequences of manmade or natural calamities such as war, civil conflict, famine, environmental depletion, and pollution. While adolescents and young people may wish to change the world as they find it, their lives have already been considerably shaped and controlled by their social environment.

It is important to recognize that every health problem has a social component. This may be the actual root of the problem (e.g., when there is malnutrition due to misconceptions about nutrition); it may consist of the reactions to a condition (e.g., what is regarded as obese in one society may be regarded as healthily plump in another); or it may be a matter of the acceptability of the potential solution to the problem (e.g., when moral strictures prevent the introduction of sex education for young people). It is difficult to conceive of any health-related problem that has no connection with the social, cultural, technological, economic, political, legal, and health and welfare systems of the society in which it occurs.

3.3 Dynamics of social change

The interaction between social factors and health issues is complex and sometimes unpredictable. For example, in Western Europe during the nineteenth century, increases in income and wealth, resulting from the Industrial Revolution, were accompanied by decreases in both birth and death rates. Many authors have in fact argued that increased income was the main cause of these changes (*13, 14*). The situation in the developing world has varied and differs from the so-called "demographic transition" in Europe. In many parts of Asia, and to a certain extent in Latin America, death rates, particularly among infants, have declined steadily in the past decade and birth rates have declined rather dramatically, yet, while there have been concomitant increases in income in many countries, these have been very modest. In Africa, on the whole, death rates (particularly of infants) remain high, birth rates are not declining, the benefits of increased income are not yet apparent, and concern over population growth is just emerging. While it has been argued that in some countries declining birth rates have helped to fuel economic growth and prosperity, in many developed and developing countries today there is concern that economic growth may be prevented by unduly low birth rates, and families are being encouraged to have more children in order to facilitate development. The relationship between wealth, birth, and death rates observed in the development of Western European countries is thus obviously not universal.

A typical feature of traditional societies is a sense of continuity and immutability in patterns of social life. Transitional societies may be better able to cope with change, and modern societies are perhaps best adapted to assimilate rapid changes. As Lengyel has argued: "Not only are modern societies pluralistic, so that innovation in one sector does not disturb the equilibrium, but they have evolved institutions to channel, order and rationalize and even induce change." (*15*).

A major difference between traditional and modern societies is that, in the former, young people can be fairly sure that their lives will be substantially similar to their parents', while, in the latter, young people can be fairly sure that their lives will be substantially different from their parents', and that their children's lives will be different from their own.

In transitional societies, young people may simultaneously be involved in two cultures: the traditional one in which their parents grew up and which they may still value, and the modern one which may be taught in schools and portrayed in the mass media. A similar clash of cultures may occur in the lives of young people whose families have migrated to another country or from a rural to an urban area.

3.4 Sources of social change affecting young people

A number of factors, the strength of which varies from culture to culture, lead to social change (*16*).

3.4.1 *General factors involved*

(*a*) *Demographic*. Changes in the number, life expectancy, and age and sex distribution of a population affecting the supply of labour and of aspirants to various social positions, affecting the degree of competition between the generations, and changing relationships between the sexes.

(*b*) *Economic*. Changes in the economic base (e.g., from primary to secondary, from secondary to tertiary), in patterns of trade, in types of property-holding, in units and modes of production, in employment or unemployment rates, in per capita income, in the percentage of gross national product spent on defence or welfare, in the distribution of income and wealth, in the exploitation of natural resources, etc.

(*c*) *Political*. Changes in patterns of authority, in access to institutions of power, in forms of government, in international alliances, etc.

(*d*) *Legal*. Changes in the legal status of minors or of women, in family law, in parental jurisdiction, in the legal availability of fertility-regulating methods, etc.

(*e*) *Religious*. Changes in the power and control of established religions, in allegiance to faiths or to sects, in relationships between organized religions and the State, in prescribed social and family roles, etc.

(*f*) *Educational.* Extension of education, changes in literacy and numeracy, in levels of investment in human skills and capital, in the pace of innovation, in the generation of social movements, etc.

(*g*) *Technological and scientific.* Changes in the complexity and efficiency of productive processes, in the efficacy of preventive and curative medicine (e.g., improved contraceptives), in desirable levels of skill, in the efficiency of communications, etc.

3.4.2 *Special problems of contemporary youth*

(*a*) *Unemployment.* Throughout the world, increasing unemployment is causing great concern. While the growth of secondary and tertiary education has often enhanced the skills of young people, opportunities to employ them are lacking (underemployment). Unemployment and underemployment are considered the most serious problems confronting young people today.

Rapid population growth has created a flood of job seekers for whom economic development is unable to create sufficient employment. Because they are the last to arrive on the labour market and lack experience, young people are the most disadvantaged when unemployment is already high, as can be seen in Table 5.

In the 24 nations of the Organization for Economic Cooperation and Development, more than 7 million young people were unemployed in 1982. In the largest countries in this group, taken together, young people accounted for around 40% of the unemployed.

In centrally planned economies, where the right to work is guaranteed by the constitution, there is no unemployment. In developing countries, where the number of young people will rise from 665 million to nearly 900 million by the end of the century, 500 million people—most of them young—are at present unemployed or underemployed. The International Labour Office estimates that 100 million jobs—88% of them in developing countries—must be created by the year 2000 for everyone to have work.

At an individual level, the emotional consequences of failing to find a job are serious and far-reaching, often resulting in despair. There is a high incidence of psychiatric disorder in young people who are unemployed, depression accounting for about 75% of the cases (*17*). Young people, women, those of lower socioeconomic status, and people already vulnerable through mental disorder are most

Table 5. Youth population and youth unemployment, 1980 (selected countries)[a]

Country or territory	Percentage of population aged 15–24	Percentage of young people unemployed
Thailand[b]	20.7	73.9
Syrian Arab Republic	20.7	69.9
India[c]	20.5	67.2
Barbados	23.2	66.2
Italy	15.2	62.4
Ghana	18.8	60.4
Venezuela[c]	21.0	58.2
Singapore	23.7	58.0
Spain[c]	16.5	57.5
Australia	17.6	55.9
Philippines[b]	21.2	54.9
Republic of Korea	23.1	48.6
Turkey[c]	21.0	48.6
Portugal	17.5	47.4
Canada	19.9	47.1
Israel	17.3	46.6
USA	18.7	45.7
Netherlands	17.2	44.7
Sweden	13.7	42.4
United Kingdom	15.8	42.2
France	15.9	42.1
Belgium	16.0	38.0
Norway	15.3	35.9
Finland	16.2	33.9
Denmark[c]	15.0	27.9
Germany, Federal Republic of	15.5	27.3
Switzerland	15.2	23.5
Japan	13.9	21.9

[a] Sources: INTERNATIONAL LABOUR OFFICE. *Report of the Director-General.* Geneva, ILO, 1982, p. 16; UNITED NATIONS. *Demographic indicators of countries: estimates and projections as assessed in 1980.* New York, United Nations, 1982.

[b] 1978.

[c] 1979.

affected by unemployment and economic recession (*18*). Suicidal behaviour is known to be significantly high among the unemployed.

The Study Group recommended that positive action be undertaken to assist unemployed young people. However, while support for the unemployed is important, it must be seen to be adequate if it is to be effective (*19*). Active research into new ways of enhancing the communication and problem-solving skills of the currently available social networks is needed in order to avoid the dangers of apathy resulting from prolonged unemployment (*20*). The development of techniques to improve leisure skills and the involvement of unemployed young people in voluntary programmes, health promotion, and social service work are examples of approaches that can be beneficial in limiting the incidence of mental disorder.

(*b*) *Migration*. Migration within and between countries can lead to social disadvantage, racial discrimination, inter-generational culture clashes, poor housing, and a lack of basic amenities, but it may also lead to greater opportunities and a higher standard of living.

(*c*) *Urbanization*. Urbanization often increases social anonymity, separation from kin, housing difficulties, pollution, crime, and unemployment. Third-world cities are experiencing very rapid population growth due to migration from rural areas. Cities like Mexico City are growing at a rate of about 12% per year. Of their rapidly increasing population, 20–25% are young people (see Fig. 5), many of whom are illiterate, unskilled, and highly vulnerable to exploitation. The result is an increased risk of homelessness, poverty, and unemployment, bringing in their wake a range of other serious problems, including drug and alcohol abuse, prostitution, violence, and poor physical and emotional health.

(*d*) *Life expectancy and health level*. Changes in life expectancy from middle age onwards have been small; the increase seen in most countries is due to the fact that a higher proportion of the population now survive infancy, childhood, and youth. Earlier maturation in respect of height, weight, and sexual development has occurred, or is occurring, in most countries. Better medical and social care in early life means that handicapped children who would have died in previous eras may now live to reach youth and adulthood (*21*). The handicapped adolescent in a transitional society is doubly disadvantaged.

(*e*) *Marriage*. Industrialization has been accompanied by a reduction in the extended family, increases in illegitimacy, divorce, and remarriage, and decreases in marriage between close kin, arranged marriages, the institution of bride price, concubinage, polygamy, fertility, and household size (*22*). In industrialized societies the average age at marriage decreased and the proportion of married people in the population increased until the early 1970s, when these trends were reversed. An increasing proportion of young people are cohabiting; there are more divorces and more remarriages of divorced people, while the proportion of marriages at which the bride is pregnant has been decreasing (*23*). Sexual mores and behaviour have become more liberal in many countries.

Fig. 5. Age and sex distribution of migrant and native populations in three cities [a, b]

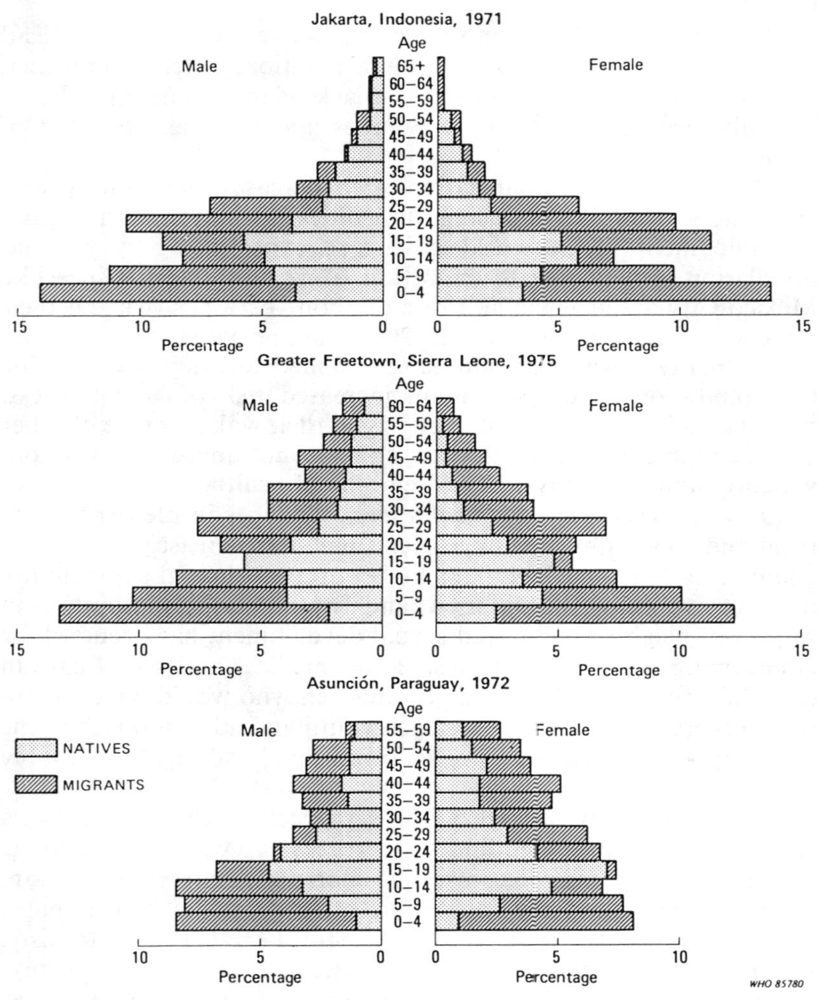

[a] Source: *Population reports. September–October 1983.* Baltimore, MD. Population Information Program, Johns Hopkins University, 1983 (Series M, No. 7), p. 257.

[b] The age and sex distribution of urban non-migrants is typical cf developing country populations with high fertility: it forms a pyramid with a broad base, indicating a high proportion of children. By contrast, most migrants are people of working ages, so their distribution is more diamond-shaped. Also, more of the migrants may be of one sex or the other, depending on the city jobs available. In Jakarta, Indonesia, as in much of Asia, men and women migrate in approximately equal numbers. In Africa, most migrants are men, as in Freetown, Sierra Leone. In the typical Latin American pattern, shown in Asuncion, Paraguay, most of the migrants are women.

(*f*) *The changing role of women.* In many countries, the status of women has been improving, creating in the process new expectations of marriage, work, and parentage, generating new demands for better access by women to educational, occupational, and political resources, and changing ideas on the propriety of such customs as female circumcision. However, some societies have sought to reverse this trend. For young people, the actual and perceived status of women is an exceedingly important factor in determining their aspirations and the timing of marriage and childbearing.

(*g*) *Communications and transport.* The increased availability of television, satellite communication, radios, telephones, motor-driven bicycles, cars, and air transport has led to an explosion in communications and travel both within and between countries. This, in turn, has resulted in a rapid spread of ideas between cultures, for better or worse, and has weakened traditional cultures. Rapidly changing attitudes among the young, changes in behaviour in certain subgroups, and a heightened degree of exploitation of the young have led to increases in sexually transmitted diseases, prostitution, and alcohol and drug abuse.

3.5 Consequences of social change

3.5.1 *Different rates of social maturation*

For more and more young people in developed and transitional societies, social maturation, i.e., the achievement of independent adult status in one's society, is being deferred. This is a consequence of the increased complexity of social structures, the need for longer periods of schooling and professional training, and the lack of employment. With earlier physical maturation, a growing number of physically mature young people are socially immature and economically dependent.

3.5.2 *Kin, community, and peer group*

The process of transition from traditional to modern societies, notably through industrialization and urbanization, has changed patterns of family formation. As a result, individuals have been removed from traditional systems of surveillance and control based on kin and community. Urban migration involving some degree of economic independence, combined with social and technological advances, has given the educated young people of today greater authority by comparison with their elders.

While peer groups, formed by the bonding together of young people of similar age, have existed as part of the cultural pattern in many traditional and tribal societies; in transitional and modern societies the rapidity of social change means that such groups may differ from their parents more than was previously the case. Ease of travel and of communications has increased the importance of young people in other societies as reference groups. Peer groups are distinguished by common life-styles which represent the ways in which they come to terms with, and solve, problems in their environment. While there is an element of choice in an individual life-style, young people are particularly prone to pressure from their peers to conform to the group's constellation of values and behaviour patterns.

3.5.3 *Stress*

In rapidly changing societies, there is a decrease in social stability leading to greater uncertainty and increasing stress by forcing choices on young people, perhaps prematurely. Another source of stress for today's young people is concern about the threats to their future presented by modern weaponry and damage to the environment.

An additional source of stress is that the rate of change is not the same in all social areas. In a changing society, changes in one sector may not keep up with changes in others, nor may different sections of the population change at the same rate. Educational systems may improve young people's skills, but they may then be underemployed. There may be investment in highly sophisticated curative medicine, while the distribution of nourishing foodstuffs to villages remains unsatisfactory. Young people may go abroad for professional education and then find themselves strangers to their families in a peasant community, where their technological skills are not applicable. Differences in the ages at which certain activities are permitted (marriage, voting, film-going, drinking, driving, consenting to medical procedures, and so on) may have confusing and ambiguous effects on young people's self-images and on their relations with others. Such inconsistencies may have adverse consequences for their health.

3.6 The effect of interacting social changes on young people's health

How such social changes (which, it must be remembered, are probably interdependent) might affect the health of young people is suggested by the model below (Fig. 6) which has been adapted from

Fig. 6. Social factors influencing the health of young people[a]

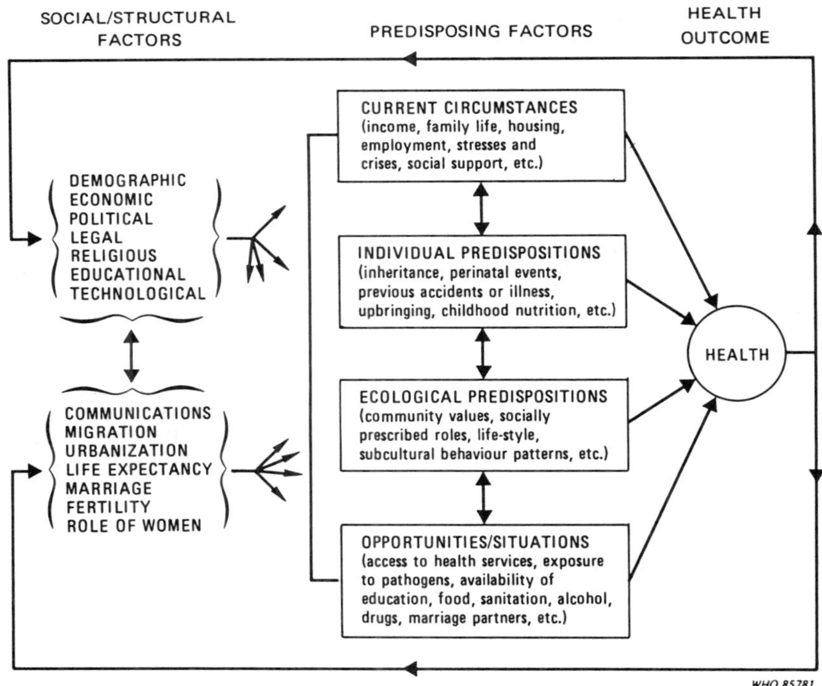

[a] Adapted from: RUTTER, M. *Changing youth in a changing society.* London, Nuffield Provincial Hospital Trust, 1978, p. 240.

one used originally to account for adolescent behaviour (*21*). This model seems equally applicable, with suitable modifications, to the health of young people, which, to a large extent, depends on their behaviour. It suggests that health is influenced by four sets of variables: individual predisposition, ecological predisposition, current circumstances, and opportunities. These variables are in turn

affected by the major sources of social change described in section
3.4.1 (the economic, political, educational, and other systems) and
by the changing patterns described in section 3.4.2. The model is a
dynamic one and shows that the health status of young people can
feed back into and influence factors relating to the social structure
which may in turn influence the predisposing variables, and
therefore health.

4. HEALTH AND HEALTH-RELATED ISSUES OF CONCERN TO YOUNG PEOPLE

4.1 The concept of health

Health is defined in the Constitution of the World Health
Organization as "a state of complete physical, mental and social
well-being" (*24*). In accepting the ambitious goal of health for all by
the year 2000, the Member States of WHO have raised important
questions as to how this can be achieved. They have also emphasized
the need to develop indicators to evaluate the progress made (*25*).

Dr H. Mahler, Director-General of WHO, suggests that health
should be considered "in the broadest context of its contribution to,
and promotion by, social and economic development, so that people
will be able to lead socially and economically satisfying lives" (*26*).
Thus, health may be seen as a state of dynamic equilibrium between
an organism and its environment.

In addition, there are important political and spiritual dimensions
to health (*27*). Powerlessness can be viewed as a basic cause of ill-
health, in that it makes individuals and communities more
vulnerable, less able to command the resources and services needed
to protect their health. A sense of helplessness may lead to passivity,
inertia, and despair.

4.2 Young people's perception of health issues

One of the earliest attempts to document the views of young
people in regard to health matters was the classic study by
Brunswick & Josephson on the health of adolescents in Harlem, New
York, USA (*28*), in which 12–15 year-olds cited drug abuse, cigarette
smoking, drinking, and insanitary living conditions (in that order)
as the most important and most threatening health problems
confronting them and their contemporaries.

A Swiss study of 930 adolescents between the ages of 16 and 19 years (*29*) reported that over 50% of the girls and 30% of the boys had noted tension and stress as being a major personal concern, whereas drug and alcohol problems rated mention by fewer than 5% of both sexes.

A comparison with similar studies reveals a high level of concordance between the results and a strong psychosocial–behavioural component (Table 6). For example, in an Australian

Table 6. Adolescents requesting help for different health problems: a cross-study comparison

	Michaud & Martin (1982) [a]	Parcel et al. (1977) [b]	Sternlieb et al. (1972) [c]	Saucier et al. (1979) [d]	Klein et al. (1981) [e]
No. in sample	930	3255	1408	277	247
Medical problems					
	(%)	(%)	(%)	(%)	(%)
acne	24	30	18	18	32
headaches	12	13	9	7	12
gynaecological (% of girls)	17	8	10	14	8
dental care	10	21	27	33	20
Psychosocial problems					
stress, anxiety	40	20	30	20	21
nutrition, weight	22	23	6	8	18
sadness, depression	20	23	–	–	24
fatigue, sleep disorders	15	16	–	–	23

[a] MICHAUD, P.A. & MARTIN, J. La santé des adolescents vaudois de 16 à 19 ans: leurs perceptions, leurs pratiques et leurs souhaits. *Revue suisse de médecine (Praxis)*, **49**: 1545–1553 (1983).

[b] PARCEL, G.S., ET AL. Adolescent health concerns, problems and patterns of utilization in a triethnic urban population. *Pediatrics*, **60**: 157–164 (1977).

[c] STERNLIEB, J.J., ET AL. A survey of health problems, practices, and needs of youth. *Pediatrics*, **49**: 177–186 (1972).

[d] SAUCIER, J.F., ET AL. Perceptions des besoins médicaux et psychologiques par les adolescents et leurs opinions sur les services. Résultats préliminaires d'une enquête. Montréal, 1980.

[e] KLEIN, D., ET AL. Comparisons between inner-city and private school adolescents' perceptions of health problems. *Journal of adolescent health care*, **3**: 82–90 (1982).

study, adolescents identified depression, getting along with parents and siblings, nervousness, making friends, acne, obesity, and development into an adult, as important issues requiring attention (N. Weston et al., unpublished observations, 1981).

The results of these investigations of adolescents' perception of health issues are interesting, since they took place in different settings and covered different socioeconomic groups (*30*). There is, however, a need for a greater involvement of young people themselves in the collection of such information, especially in developing countries where differences of outlook related to cultural factors may be expected.

Where migrations of the young occur, there is a special need to learn more about the effects of exposure to "mixed" values and to transmit this information to professional health care workers.

4.3 Problems of classification

Health needs have been described as a "composite of multiple complex factors which in sum define a series of normative reference standards" (*31*). A number of considerations have to be taken into account: adolescents are not a homogeneous group and various intra-group differences will have implications for health needs; the needs of boys and girls vary, as do those of early, middle, and late adolescents; an individual's personal potential, immediate environment, and the presence or absence of certain risk factors are all relevant; at a broader level, national, social, and cultural differences markedly influence health needs.

A variety of approaches have been suggested (*32*). The listing of problems, even within several broad categories, is of relatively limited value at an international level, because of a lack of available data and problems of comparability. Furthermore, "pure" health issues cannot usefully be separated from health-related issues such as unemployment, income maintenance, housing, transport, and socioeconomic status. But it is possible to identify problems that afflict large numbers of young people and are specific to their particular age groups. While some conditions exist in both developing and developed countries, others are related to the degree of development.

The health needs of young people must therefore be studied in widely differing circumstances, taking into account the various factors noted above. These factors, as well as the interrelationship between the biological, psychological, and social aspects of health, have made it difficult to classify the health issues and problems relevant to young people. Nevertheless, a variety of approaches have been suggested. For the purposes of this report, the following categories have been chosen for discussion: life-style and risk-taking behaviour; emotional and related problems; sexual and reproductive health; and biological and medical problems.

4.4 Life-style and risk-taking behaviour

4.4.1 *The concept of life-style*

For the past three decades, research into the health of young people and the planning of appropriate services and health education have had a strong behavioural orientation which is best understood in the context of individual life-styles.

Life-styles may be defined as mediating structures reflecting a whole range of social values, attitudes, and activities. An individual's choice of behaviour may be either health-promoting or detrimental to health. To modify a young person's life-style, however, comprehensive measures are required to change the factors that determine it.[1]

While an individual may change a specific type of behaviour, it is less easy for him (or her) to change his (or her) reference group, and its influences always remain very important. For this reason programmes to change behaviour that do not take the reference group into account are likely to fail. As life-styles tend to be enduring, a long-term approach is required for change.

Health is both a consequence of an individual's life-style and a factor in determining it but it cannot be isolated from other aspects of life.

4.4.2 *Behaviour patterns and health*

The life-styles of young people usually involve greater risk-taking behaviour than those of other groups in the population. Smoking, alcohol and drug abuse, and disregard of traffic regulations are examples of behaviour patterns that frequently endanger young people's health. Their alteration is, therefore, the principal aim of trials being carried out in both developing and developed countries. Educational measures to encourage young people to break away from behaviour patterns carrying a health risk, or to "immunize" young adolescents against them, have tended to have moderate, short-term effects only, with no marked success in the long term.

Risk-taking is, however, a natural part of growing up. In a longitudinal study of American adolescents, Jessor & Jessor discovered that "breaking away from abstinence" is an integral part

---

[1] *Intervention studies related to life-styles conducive to health: report on a workshop.* Copenhagen, WHO Regional Office for Europe, 1983 (unpublished document ICP/HED/019(3)/12).

of the process of forming an individual, socially acceptable life-style and relating it to everyday life (*33*). While risk-taking behaviour may constitute a health hazard, it often simultaneously provides a young person with a sense of "adultness".

In Europe, according to the Projektgruppe Jugendbüro (*34*), for lower- and middle-class adolescents aged 12 years and over, smoking, drinking, and visiting pubs are as important as making friends or gaining sexual experience. They may even be pivotal to the adolescent's self-respect. They are ways of taking part in what are perceived as adult activities, even if only symbolically. Risk-taking behaviour may also offer young people a means of escape from the resolution of personal conflicts. The benefits may thus be short-term, while the harm done can be lasting.

Among young people, opportunities for risk-taking behaviour seem to be increasing. Without wider changes in society, the provision of health information is insufficient in itself to reduce the prevalence of behaviour dangerous to health. Programmes aimed at reducing risk-taking behaviour should encompass (*35*):

—risk experience and experimentation;
—risk awareness;
—risk assessment;
—risk control.

Another approach, that of "psychological" immunization against risk-taking behaviour (analogous to immunizing infants against infectious diseases to which they are especially vulnerable), is still in its infancy and needs development and evaluation.

4.4.3 *Smoking*

Cigarette smoking has been characterized repeatedly as "one of the greatest health hazards of modern times" (*36*) as well as the major cause of avoidable death. Young people who take up smoking have been shown to experience an early onset of cough, phlegm production, and shortness of breath on exertion (*37*). There is evidence from the USA that the earlier a person begins to smoke, the greater the risk of life-threatening diseases such as chronic bronchitis, emphysema, cardiovascular disease, and lung cancer (*38*).

Smoking, with its accompanying effects on health, has until recently been mainly a concern of developed countries.[1] In some of which there have been significant decreases in the numbers of young smokers, e.g., Canada, Sweden, and the USA (Fig. 7). Table 7

Fig. 7. Trends in the prevalence of cigarette smoking among boys and girls in the USA[a]

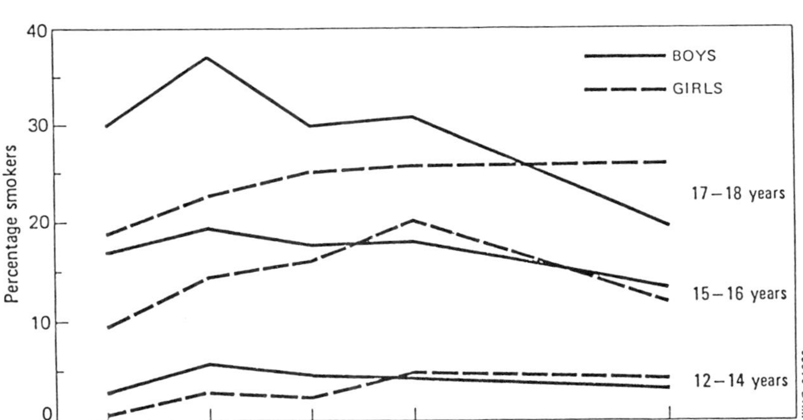

[a]Source: MASIRONI, R. & ROY, L. *Cigarette smoking in young age groups. Geographic prevalence.* Geneva, World Health Organization (unpublished document WHO/SMO/82.3).

shows the prevalence of smoking by young people in selected countries. Smoking by girls has increased to such an extent that, in some developed countries, more girls smoke than boys. In those developing countries where tobacco companies have undertaken aggressive marketing campaigns, long-range trends suggest an impending epidemic (*39*). Also, it is notable that in developing countries the habit of smoking is acquired at a very early age.

Experimentation with smoking as a symbol of "adult" behaviour is common in adolescence. The literature suggests that three factors are associated with young people smoking: peer pressure, following the example of siblings and parents, and employment outside the home. Data from the USA suggest that, if a child's older sibling and

---

[1] MASIRONI, R. & ROY, L. *Smoking in developing countries.* Geneva, WHO International Clearing-house on Smoking and Health Information, 1983 (unpublished document WHO/SMO/83.1), p. 1.

Table 7. Prevalence of smoking among young people [a]

Country or territory	Year	Age group (years)	Percentage who smoke	
			females	males
Argentina (La Plata)	1971–2	15–24	31	57
Brazil (São Paulo)	1971–2	15–24	20	54
Bulgaria	1975	15–17	30	79
Chile (Santiago)	1971–2	15–24	30	50
Colombia (Bogotá)	1971–2	15–24	15	51
Denmark	1976	15–19	42	35
Egypt	1982 [b]	10–19	0.2	7
Ethiopia (Gondar)	1978	12–23	3	28
Germany, Federal Republic of	1976	14–19	40	41
Greece	– [c]	15–18	54	46
Guatemala (Guatemala City)	1971–2	15–24	5	24
India (Delhi)	1978 [b]	12–19	4	10
Italy	1972	15–18	55	51
Kuwait	1980 [b]	20–24	7	44
Mexico (Mexico City)	1971–2	15–24	12	35
Netherlands	1981	15–19	30	27
New Zealand	1976	12–16	30	30
Nigeria (Lagos)	1974	13–18	5	17
Peru (Lima)	1971–2	15–24	5	24
Senegal (Dakar)	1980 [b]	10–20	52	71
Sri Lanka (Colombo)	1975–6	15–20	– [c]	12
Switzerland	1975	18–20	46	36
United Kingdom	1980	16–19	37	42
Venezuela (Caracas)	1971–2	15–24	25	39

[a] Adapted from: MASIRONI, R. & ROY, L. Cigarette smoking in young age groups. Geographic prevalence. Geneva, World Health Organization (unpublished document WHO/SMO/82.3); and MASIRONI, R. & ROY, L. Smoking in developing countries. Geneva, World Health Organization, 1982 (unpublished document WHO/SMO/83.1).

[b] Year data published.

[c] Not available.

both parents smoke, the child is four times as likely to smoke as one with no smoking model in the family (*40*). For measures to deal with the problems associated with smoking, refer to Sections 5 and 6.

4.4.4 *Alcohol consumption*

Over the past 30–40 years, increasing percentages of children and adolescents have started to drink alcoholic beverages, their alcohol consumption has increased in quantity and frequency, and the age at which drinking starts has declined (*41*). This situation is disturbing because the young people concerned may run a greater risk of alcohol problems in later life and also, in the short term, because of increased rates of drunkenness and involvement in road accidents.

The populations at greatest risk appear to be those in areas undergoing rapid sociocultural and economic change where cultural controls on overindulgence are breaking down and alcohol is becoming increasingly available. Social and environmental factors are known to be important in the development of drinking among the young, a crucial role being played by parents and peers. Disadvantaged young people are particularly at risk. The consequences for individuals include under-attainment of developmental tasks, social decline, educational loss, and unemployment.

Young people's attitudes to alcohol are significant. Data on a sample of young people at high schools in the USA showed that those labelled as "problem drinkers" tended to place a lower value on conventional goals, were more tolerant towards "transgression behaviours", and had greater social support for drinking than those not labelled "problem drinkers" (*42*).

Similarities in research data from several different countries suggest (*42*) that the images and beliefs associated with drinking in young people are generally much the same. Given the probable cross-national character of certain features of the social environment relevant to alcohol consumption by young people, the processes whereby learned symbolic values become attached to alcohol consumption should be of international concern.

Some of the health problems of those who drink heavily, even if not alcohol-dependent, are summarized below (*43*).

—*Consequences of an acute episode of heavy drinking:*
  short-term impairment of functioning and control;
  aggressiveness; accidents; exposure to climatic conditions;
  physical disorders; arrest for drunkenness.

—*Consequences of prolonged heavy drinking:*
  cirrhosis of the liver; aggravation of other physical disorders;
  malnutrition; prolonged impairment of functioning and control;
  accidents; impairment of working capacity;
  alcohol dependence syndrome; alcoholic psychosis.

—*Possible concomitants:*
  loss of friends, family, health, self-esteem, job, means of support,
  and liberty.

4.4.5 *Use and abuse of drugs*

The average age of drug users has decreased considerably in recent years. Multiple drug-use has also become more common. The problem exists in virtually all societies and socioeconomic groups. Some of the social and environmental factors associated with a high risk for drug abuse are listed in Table 8.

Table 8. Factors associated with a high risk for drug abuse[a]

– unemployment	– areas where drugs are sold, traded, or produced
– living away from home	
– migration to cities	– certain occupations (tourism, drug production or sale)
– relaxed parental control	
– alienation from family	– areas with high rates of crime or vice
– early exposure to drugs	
– leaving school early	– areas where there are drug-using gangs
– poor use of drugs	
– broken homes; one-parent families	– areas where delinquency is common
– large urban environments	

[a] Adapted from SMART, R.G., ET AL. *Drug use among non-student youths.* Geneva, World Health Organization, 1981, pp. 10–11 (WHO Offset Publication No. 60).

Drug-taking reflects self-destructiveness, but may also be a form of social protest. Concern over drug-use by teenagers increased in the late 1960s, particularly in the developed countries. A survey of data from 33 countries around 1970 *(44)* yielded the following figures: in the Netherlands, 11.15% of secondary school children had experimented with drugs once (2.5% more than 20 times); in Sweden, 8% of the ninth grade students (4% more than 10 times) and 6% of university students (5% more than once); Switzerland, 19.6% of a representative sample of young people aged 13–20 years had used drugs "at least once" (4.7% had used them "often").

Cannabis emerged in the late 1960s as the drug (apart from alcohol) most widely used for nonmedical purposes, particularly in the younger age groups.

Evidence of the use of other drugs to varying degrees is provided by the data from Canada, India, Malaysia, and Pakistan presented in Table 9.

In countries with long experience of heavy drug use, there is a tendency to prefer a single drug, perhaps because a continuous supply is less problematic. Multiple drug use may be more common where drug abuse is a relatively recent occurrence. In a number of countries, the sniffing of substances such as glue, petrol, and other

Table 9. Percentage of persons having used specific kinds of drug at any time or within the preceding 12 months: data from four centres[a]

Drug (group)	Chandigarh (n = 393)		Islamabad (n = 360)		Penang (n = 90)		Toronto (n = 430)	
	Any time	Last 12 months	Any time	Last 12 months	Any time	Last 12 months	Any time	Last 12 months
cannabis	3.1	2.0	84.4	83.9	2.2	0.0	51.2	35.1
amphetamines	1.0	0.3	0.3	0.3	3.3	1.1	9.5	4.4
barbiturates/ sedatives	–	–	6.7	6.4	3.3	1.1	6.3	2.6
hallucinogens	–	–	0.3	0.0	–	–	15.4	6.1
cocaine	–	–	0.3	0.3	–	–	6.3	1.6
opium	3.6	2.3	13.1	12.2	0.0	0.0	4.4	1.9

– Items not used.

[a] Adapted from SMART, R.G., ET AL. *Drug use among non-students.* Geneva, World Health Organization, 1981, p. 22 (WHO Offset Publication No. 60).

volatile chemicals is causing increasing concern, as it can result in death, even on the first occasion. In chronic abusers, damage to the brain, the peripheral nervous system, the kidneys, the liver, or the heart may occur, depending on the solvent used (*45*).

The causes of drug dependence are usually numerous. Experimentation and risk-taking, so characteristic of the young, figure prominently in the reasons for which drugs are initially used. For example, research into the reasons for drug abuse among university students in India yielded the following: 61.6% used drugs out of curiosity on an experimental basis; 31.6% for "kicks"; and 32.4% to help deal with problems, stresses, and failures (*46*). While only some users stay with the practice, the risk of chronic dependence needs no stressing.

4.4.6 *Accidents*

Accidents constitute one of the major causes of death in adolescence throughout the world (Table 10), accounting in many countries for about half of all deaths in the age group 10–24 years. Moreover, particularly in developing countries, their importance as a cause of death is increasing. Besides costing lives, accidents leave many disabled and maimed. While some accidents may be said to be wholly accidental in that there was no predisposing behaviour (e.g., if someone is struck by a brick falling from a roof), many have a behavioural component that may increase the risk of a harmful outcome (e.g., not wearing protective clothing at work). When there

Table 10. Accidents as a proportion of all causes of death among persons aged 10–24 years in certain countries, by WHO Region (latest available figures)[a]

Region and country or territory	Year	%	Region and country or territory	Year	%
Africa			Denmark	1980	47.3
Mauritius	1981	39.4	Finland	1978	37.0
			France	1978	54.0
Americas			Germany, Federal Republic of	1980	53.3
Canada	1978	56.8	Greece	1980	52.0
Chile	1979	16.2	Hungary	1980	36.5
Costa Rica	1979	43.2	Italy	1978	50.0
Dominican Republic	1978	18.0	Netherlands	1980	46.5
El Salvador	1974	20.6	Norway	1980	51.8
Mexico	1976	21.2	Spain	1979	50.9
Panama	1974	31.0	Sweden	1980	40.8
Paraguay	1977	21.5	Switzerland	1980	47.9
Puerto Rico	1977	35.1	United Kingdom		
Trinidad	1977	35.1	England and Wales	1980	45.9
USA	1978	54.5	Northern Ireland	1978	54.8
Uruguay	1978	40.2	Scotland	1981	52.0
Venezuela	1978	45.8	Yugoslavia	1979	45.2
Eastern Mediterranean			**South-East Asia**		
Egypt	1978	12.3	Thailand	1980	19.9
Israel [b]	1980	34.2			
			Western Pacific		
Europe			Australia	1980	63.3
Austria	1980	53.9	Hong Kong	1981	35.0
Bulgaria	1981	39.4	Japan	1980	36.0
Czechoslovakia	1975	46.5	Singapore	1981	25.2

[a] From information available to WHO.

[b] Editors' footnote. It was resolved by the Thirty-eighth World Health Assembly in May 1985 that Israel shall form part of the WHO European Region.

are related behavioural components accidents are often preventable. Because of the propensity of young people to take risks, this is an area requiring particular attention.

While older people may indulge in behaviour that has adverse consequences in the longer term—choosing a bad diet (where there is a choice) or being overly sedentary—it is more characteristic of young people to indulge in dangerous behaviour involving an immediate risk, e.g., recklessness in traffic, experimenting with drugs, taking unnecessary chances in sports or at work, or having unprotected sexual intercourse when a pregnancy would be unwelcome. While road accidents involving young people may be due to factors beyond the individual's control, such as poor roads, other factors such as impulsiveness, carelessness about safety measures, and drinking or drug-taking while driving are preventable (*47*). It is also likely that a proportion of "accidents" may actually be disguised suicides, albeit this is very difficult to assess.

The young adolescent, of course, lacks life experience and needs supervision to ensure that he or she exercises some degree of caution. Again, the more young people participate in activities that provide them with healthy outlets involving some measure of personal choice, the more they will learn to assume individual responsibility and to cooperate with others. In sports and entertainment, exemplary behaviour by respected figures can be invaluable in the prevention of accidents.

While a number of individual factors increase the danger of accidents during adolescence, including impulsiveness, risk-taking, curiosity, experimentation with "adult" ways, and, in a minority of cases, pathological self-destructive behaviour, there are also societal influences that can be reduced, notably access to dangerous substances, advertising encouraging hazardous activities, hazards in the working environment, and inadequate safety legislation.

Advances in technology have made it possible to devise more effective programmes to reduce some of the environmental risk factors indicated in Table 11. Examples of successful measures include the safety packaging of medicaments and changes in the minimum drinking and driving ages (*48*).

4.5 Emotional problems

While emotional difficulties can, of course, be experienced at any time of life, adolescents are subject to special stresses arising from the rapid changes that accompany their transition from childhood to adulthood. In addition, as a result of the transitional state of many societies today, external stresses are brought to bear on young people. These stresses, and the ways in which young people cope with them need to be understood for at least two major reasons: while the experience of stress is a natural part of maturation, it can, if not dealt with in a healthy way, lead to emotional and physical disorders with serious consequences for both individuals and families; at the same time, adolescence provides an opportunity for helping young people to learn how to cope and thus achieve a healthy future for themselves and their future families.

Table 11. Factors influencing risk-taking behaviour by adolescents with regard
to accidents

Individual factors	Environmental factors
– Increase in aggressiveness and impulsiveness during puberty (hormone-based)	– Tacit or overt acceptance of certain behaviour by family (e.g., the "tough athlete" may reflect exaggerated ideas of parental requirements or wishes)
– Impaired perception of risks (related to stage of cognitive development)	– Seeking peer approval or submitting to peer pressure (i.e., the need to belong is a powerful motivation to behave in certain ways)
– Tendency to behave contrary to family or social expectations (as part of striving for self-determination)	– Societal factors, including the availability of dangerous things (e.g., motor cars); media influence (advertising of substances and products open to abuse, as well as sexual innuendos and the general glorification of violence)
– Curiosity and experimentation (or a relatively normal degree of youthful exuberance)	– Physical environment (including workplace, traffic patterns)
– For a minority of individuals, dangerous behaviour may be motivated by other psychological factors: e.g., "counter-phobic" behaviour (doing what is actually feared but with the fear repressed or denied); dangerous behaviour as a manifestation of underlying suicidal wishes	– Legislative factors (seat-belt and helmet laws, import laws, minimum driving age)

4.5.1 Sources of stress

Two major sources of stress, individual and societal, are described
below.

(a) *Individual*. The transitional period between the dependence of
childhood and the independence of adulthood is characterized by
continual change. During this time adolescents form deep
attachments with others of their own age and feel painful emotional
experiences very keenly. Uncertainties about their own identity and
what the future will bring come to the fore. The need to compete with
their peers and, at the same time, to win social approval are both
very strong and often place individuals in situations of extreme
conflict. The need for parental approval coexists with the need to
achieve a degree of independence. The strength of the sexual drive
increases, while, at the same time, social taboos concerning
behaviour are intensified. There is a need to express oneself as an
individual side-by-side with a strong pull towards conformity to the
peer group. Some of the powerful feelings thus created are being
experienced for the first time and may lead to a certain
bewilderment. All these factors, and others, combine to create
stresses for which adolescents may not be fully prepared. Most will

cope with the changes in themselves and the new types of behaviour now expected of them, but some will react to stress in an unhealthy way and develop neurotic or psychotic conditions for which they will need help.

(*b*) *Societal.* A second major source of stress for contemporary adolescents, particularly in transitional societies, is the conflict generated by new opportunities and new frustrations arising from societal changes. These stress-inducing conditions include: the wave of migration from rural to urban or periurban areas and the consequent diminution in the traditional family support system; a greater exposure, through the entertainment media, to ideas that had previously been culturally alien; tourism; the migration of other citizens to and from foreign countries; changes in the technological needs of society requiring skills that are different from those of the previous generation and for which the training or education available may be inadequate; the encouragement by commercial interests of economic aspirations that are often unrealistic; and economic injustices and threats to peace created by international factors that the young feel powerless to control. All of these factors, separately and together, place stress on contemporary youth. The pressure is mostly felt where young people have little control over their own destinies, where rapid population expansion means greater competition in the younger age groups, and where resources are inadequate to meet their needs.

The combined effect of these two types of modern stress—the individual and the societal—makes it imperative to take steps to prevent damage to the young and to facilitate the use of the positive qualities of adolescence in ways that are both healthy for young people and of value to their communities.

4.5.2 *Health implications of stress*

It is well understood that the causation of physical and psychological disorders is multifactoral. Psychological stress and inadequate coping ability contribute to illness (*49*). The experience of stress, particularly in the absence of a social support system or when there is a discrepancy between the actual and perceived demands of a stressful situation, may contribute to further disorders, as in the transactional model suggested by Lazarus & Cohen (*50*). The interaction between stress, coping, and disease has been of long-standing interest to clinicians. Psychological stress has been

implicated as a contributory factor in virtually all diseases (*51*). In
particular, there are direct links between stress and hypertension and
coronary heart disease.

Stress, if not dealt with properly, may be the cause of accidents
as well as illness. When there is pressure on workers to be productive,
they may become careless about avoiding occupational hazards or
using protective devices. Young workers, lacking experience and
grateful to find employment when times are hard, may be
particularly vulnerable. The need to achieve social status with peers
will sometimes result in substance abuse, which, in turn, will make
accidents more likely. In modern or transitional societies, social
pressures that encourage unprotected sexual activity make young
people more vulnerable to sexually transmitted diseases, to
unwanted pregnancies, and to risky induced abortions.

4.5.3 *High-risk groups*

Among the younger members of the population, the following
subgroups are likely to contain individuals who are more vulnerable
than their peers (*52*):

—racial, religious, or ethnic minorities;
—those who have experienced significant loss, including
  bereavement, disrupted homes, or parental rejection; those in
  institutional care;
—those suffering from physical or intellectual impairment due to
  chronic illness and/or disability;
—those whose parents suffer from chronic physical or mental
  illness;
—victims of physical, emotional, or sexual abuse;
—the homeless, the unemployed, the very poor;
—pregnant adolescents and teenage parents.

4.5.4 *Coping behaviour*

The acquisition of adaptive strategies to cope with stress may
limit the incidence of maladaptive behaviour and avert eventual
illness. Adaptive strategies also provide early relief from stress and
enhance self-reliance when the subject is exposed to further stress
factors. The needs in this area include:

(*a*) improved identification of stress factors by techniques that could help young people to perceive, predict, and understand them;

(*b*) the promotion of problem-solving strategies by training young people to pose and define problems and learn how to establish a range of solutions;

(*c*) the training of young people in emotion-regulating processes by helping them to identify and understand their emotions and to display and verbalize them in socially acceptable ways;

(*d*) the provision of guidance on forms of direct action that can avoid exposure to stress factors or readily dissipate their effects;

(*e*) training in techniques for effective communication in situations of stress and when anticipating stress factors.

4.5.5 *Psychiatric disorders*

Although adolescents are subject to special stress, well-documented studies from the United Kingdom and the USA have, in the past decade, refuted the notion that continuous psychological turmoil is universal and normal for adolescents (*11*). Although almost 50% of young people report some significant stress during their teenage years, the prevalence of significant psychiatric disorders in adolescents is believed to be between 12% and 15%.

The assessment of what is normal and what is abnormal in adolescent behaviour can be difficult, but certain warning signs can suggest the need for expert evaluation and help. These include poor peer relationships, frequent or prolonged mood disturbance, chronic hyperactivity, isolation, psychosomatic symptoms, a poor self-image, and repeated antisocial acts.

Psychological disturbance ranges from stress-induced emotional problems of a minor and transitory nature to serious psychiatric disorders. Treatment should seek, where possible, not only to help disturbed adolescents, individually, but also to involve their families.

4.5.6 *Suicidal behaviour*

Evidence from the USA shows that suicides among young people have risen markedly in the past two decades, making it the third leading cause of death. The overall rate of attempted suicide has also been steadily increasing, the increase being greatest and the rates highest among young people (*53*). Furthermore, the ratio of attempted suicide to successful suicide has been estimated at 100 : 1.

Many deaths recorded as accidental are believed to be disguised suicides. All in all, suicidal behaviour constitutes an alarming and growing problem among young people.

Suicide is underreported for a number of reasons, and, while the reliability of the statistics may be affected by variations in the definition and reporting of cases, studies suggest that sources of error are sufficiently random to permit comparisons between countries (*54*).

Suicide rates among 10–24-year-olds in selected countries are shown in Table 12 for 1973 and the latest available year. It can be noted that in the many of these countries, there has been an increase in the rates.

The reasons for suicidal behaviour are complex and not always clear; however, it is usually associated with feelings of depression, loss, and hopelessness, often resulting from frustration. Stress arising from rapid social change, decreasing family stability, confused values, and, in particular, unemployment, undoubtedly contribute to suicidal impulses. Attempted suicide rates are highest in poor urban areas, where other indices of social disorganization are high. Individuals who have suffered from depression, who have experienced suicide in the family, or who have previously attempted suicide are at particularly high risk.

The early detection of adolescents who might attempt suicide should focus on the identification of depressive illness, the evaluation of signs of alienation, and the perception of mounting anxiety (*55*). Secondary prevention should be undertaken where there is high risk, and should aim at improving the future prospects of the individual concerned. Programmes for the prevention of suicide in young people might usefully involve families, peer groups, and community leaders, as well as professional personnel.

4.6 Sexual and reproductive health

4.6.1 *General situation*

While data on adolescent sexuality and fertility are still inadequate, particularly in developing countries, biomedical and psychosocial studies in a number of countries have been stimulated by the WHO Task Force on Reproductive Health in Adolescence.

While the situation in no two countries is identical, three patterns of sexual and reproductive behaviour can be broadly distinguished:

Table 12. Suicide rates per 100 000 population among persons aged 10–24 years in certain countries, by WHO Region (1973 and latest available figures)[a]

Region and country or territory	Year	Rate	Region and country or territory	Year	Rate
Africa			Finland	1978	14.4
Mauritius	1981	0.9		1973	15.8
	1973	7.4	France	1978	6.7
				1973	5.3
Americas			Germany, Federal	1980	8.0
Canada	1978	12.1	Republic of	1973	8.0
	1973	8.4	Greece	1980	1.5
Chile	1979	5.1		1973	1.5
	1973	4.4	Hungary	1980	14.8
Costa Rica	1979	2.7		1973	12.0
	1973	2.1	Italy	1978	2.2
Dominican Republic	1978	2.0		1973	1.9
	1973	3.2	Netherlands	1980	4.1
El Salvador	1974	16.9		1973	3.6
	1973	12.6	Norway	1980	8.4
Mexico	1976	2.1		1973	3.5
	1973	0.7	Poland	1980	–
Panama	1974	2.4		1973	8.2
	1972	3.5	Portugal	1979	5.0
Paraguay	1977	4.7		1973	–
	1973	3.4	Spain	1979	1.9
Puerto Rico	1977	4.4		1973	1.0
	1973	4.5	Sweden	1980	7.7
Trinidad	1977	8.9		1973	10.5
	1973	8.9	Switzerland	1980	16.4
USA	1978	8.8		1973	9.4
	1973	7.2	United Kingdom		
Uruguay	1978	6.2	England and Wales	1980	3.2
	1973	7.0		1973	2.9
Venezuela	1978	4.8	Northern Ireland	1978	2.8
	1973	5.4		1973	2.5
			Scotland	1981	4.9
Eastern Mediterranean				1973	3.5
Egypt	1978	0.2	Yugoslavia	1979	5.9
	1973	0.1		1973	–
Israel[b]	1980	3.9			
	1973	3.2	**South-East Asia**		
			Thailand	1980	10.6
Europe				1973	6.2
Austria	1980	13.3			
	1973	8.1	**Western Pacific**		
Bulgaria	1981	5.2	Australia	1980	7.6
	1973	4.9		1973	7.0
Czechoslovakia	1975	11.4	Hong Kong	1981	4.7
	1973	12.6		1973	6.4
Denmark	1980	8.2	Japan	1980	8.2
	1973	6.1		1973	11.9
			Singapore	1981	4.2
				1973	6.4

– Data not available.

[a] From information available to WHO.

[b] It was resolved by the Thirty-eighth World Health Assembly in May 1985 that Israel shall form part of the WHO European Region.

(*a*) The first, which is found mainly in developed countries, is characterized by the onset of sexual experience in the mid–late teens, a low use of contraceptives, a high incidence of unwanted nonmarital pregnancy, a demonstrable tendency for recourse to abortion (largely legal and relatively safe), late marriage, low fertility, significant rates of sexually transmitted disease, and undesirable rates of sexual violence.

(*b*) The second pattern (almost the direct opposite) is characterized by marriage at an age corresponding, more or less, with menarche and early frequent childbearing, with a consequent high rate of population growth. Premarital sexual activity is uncommon, as is premarital pregnancy or childbirth. Contraception is rare, and abortion is usually illegal and unsafe. In some areas there is a high incidence of sexually transmitted disease with subsequent infertility because of inadequate health care.

(*c*) The third pattern, found particularly in urban settings in transitional societies, occupies a middle ground. Sexual as well as educational and economic opportunities are expanding for youth, especially women. Patterns of fertility and sexuality are transitional and somewhat mixed. The traditional social restraints are still largely evident but less effective than in the past, the age of marriage is rising, premarital sex and pregnancy are increasing among the young, as is recourse to abortion, and overall fertility is beginning to decline as contraception is used more and more.

The wide variation in patterns of marriage and fertility can be seen from Table 13 and Fig. 8. Further examples of changing patterns are given below.

Though the minimum legal age of marriage in Tunisia is 17 years, by 1975 the mean age of marriage for women had risen to 23.3 years. In certain areas of Nigeria, premarital sexual activity is on the increase, as is the use of contraception. A survey in Ibadan in 1983 indicated that three-quarters of unmarried males and one-half of unmarried females aged 14–25 years were sexually active and that two-thirds of them had used contraception (the rate being roughly four times higher than the national rate). Of the group of females, nearly 50% had had at least one pregnancy, terminated in most instances by abortion. In other parts of Nigeria, on the other hand, marriage takes place very early, and fertility is high and welcomed. In developing countries generally, contraception is rarely practised by adolescents.

Table 13. Percentage of younger women who are married, by age group
(selected countries)[a]

Country or territory	Age group		
	10–14 (%)	15–19 (%)	20–24 (%)
Bangladesh	8.2	64.7	91.0
Indonesia	0.8	24.6	66.2
Mexico	–	17.7	56.6
Pakistan	1.3	37.4	75.3
Peru	–	14.5	49.0
Republic of Korea	–	3.2	43.6
Sri Lanka	–	6.2	37.8

– Data not available.

[a] Reproduced, by permission, from: KABIR, M. *The demographic characteristics of household populations*. London, World Fertility Survey, 1980 (Comparative Studies, Cross-National Summaries, No. 6).

The age of first sexual intercourse appears to be declining; a recent survey in Europe indicated that at the age of 18 years 50% of males and 33% of females have had sexual experience. Earlier menarche, cultural factors, socioeconomic conditions, and the status of women influence the differences between the figures for boys and those for girls (Table 14). Also, with increasingly permissive social attitudes, young people are subjected to more peer-group pressure to be sexually active. Throughout the world teenagers are being bombarded with sexual images and innuendoes by the media. An important example of this is the way advertising suggests a link, especially in the case of young women, between smoking and sexual attractiveness. Nevertheless, it should be noted that most sexually active teenagers have intercourse infrequently, and that relatively few have intercourse with more than one or two partners. In general, sexually active young people tend to be discriminating and basically monogamous, particularly during the later years of adolescence. In virtually every area of sexual and reproductive activity young people are particularly exposed to certain health risks, some of which are outlined below.

4.6.2 *Pregnancy, abortion, and childbirth*

Pregnancy in adolescence, particularly in the younger age groups, is associated with greater mortality and morbidity, among both mothers (Tables 15 and 16) and offspring (Tables 17 and 18). Table 16 shows not only that the maternal mortality rate is highest among

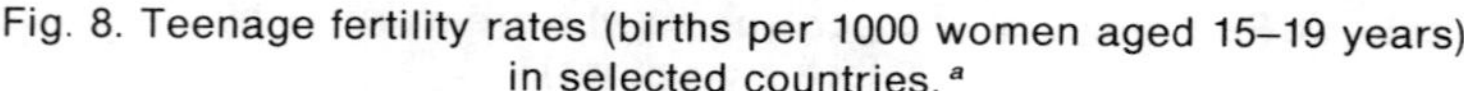

Fig. 8. Teenage fertility rates (births per 1000 women aged 15–19 years) in selected countries. [a]

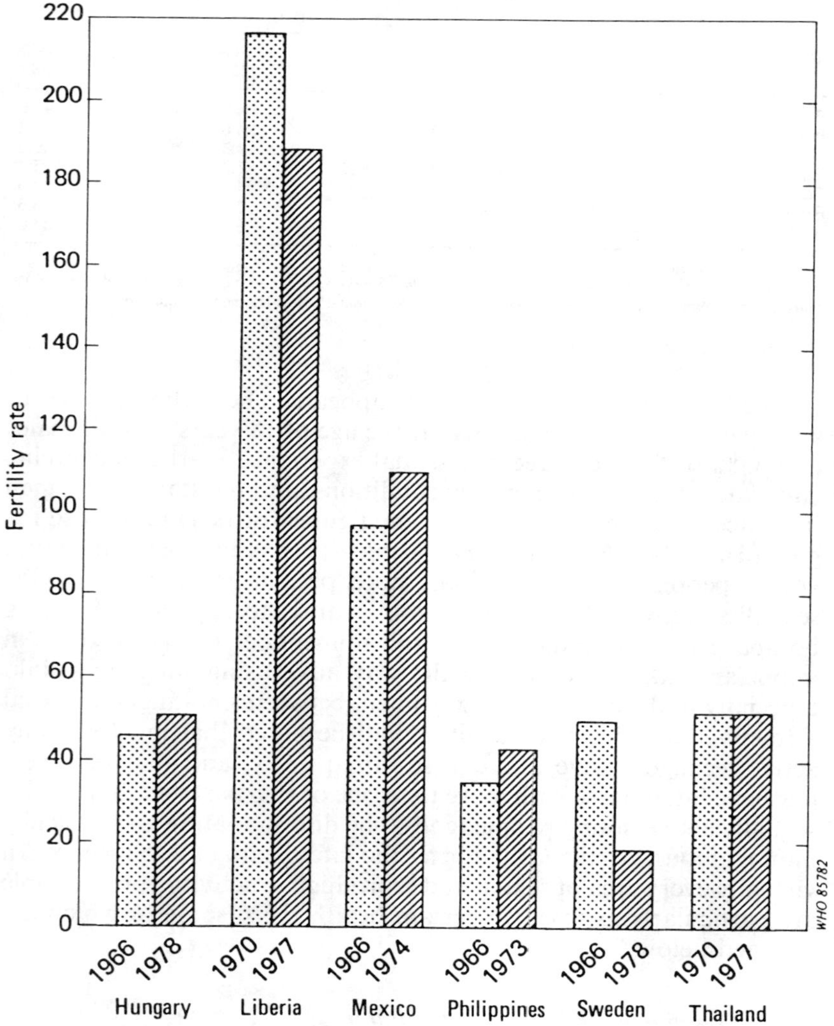

[a] Sources: *UN demographic yearbook* and other information available to WHO.

Table 14. Percentage of adolescents reported to have experienced premarital coitus (selected countries)

Country or territory	Age range (years)	Percentage sexually experienced	
		Males	Females
Australia	By age 20	58	47
Germany, Federal Republic of	By age 16	35	30
Israel	14–19	42	11
Japan	16–21	15	7
Nigeria	14–19	68	43
Republic of Korea	12–21	17	4

[a] Adapted from HOFMANN, A.D. Contraception in adolescence: A review. 1. Psychological aspects. *Bulletin of the World Health Organization*, **62**: 151–162 (1984).

Table 15. Age-specific maternal mortality rates (selected countries)[a]

Country or territory	Year	Maternal deaths per 10 000 live births	
		15–19 years	20–24 years
Australia	1975	1.4	6.9
Dominican Republic	1976	129.9	59.1
Ecuador	1976	202.7	141.3
England and Wales	1977	10.5	6.3
France	1977	12.3	13.8
Greece	1977	10.0	8.1
Japan	1978	29.5	14.4
Malaysia (peninsular)	1977	91.3	56.2
Netherlands	1976	6.1	5.8
Thailand	1977	103.9	86.8
USA	1975	7.7	8.6
Venezuela	1977	45.4	41.3
Yugoslavia	1977	18.1	12.0

[a] Source: WORLD HEALTH ORGANIZATION. *Report of a WHO meeting on adolescent sexuality and reproductive health: educational and service aspects, Mexico, 1980.* Geneva, 1981 (unpublished WHO document MCH/RHA 81.1).

the very young, but also that antenatal care is associated with a reduction in maternal mortality in all age groups. Furthermore, although this is not shown in the table, young women are less likely than older women to receive antenatal care.

The most common problems are anaemia, retardation of fetal growth, premature birth, and complications of labour (56). Repeated pregnancies in the adolescent period increase future risks to reproductive health. In addition, the children of adolescent mothers are more likely to be exposed to illness and injury. Pregnancy in a still-growing girl means an increase in nutritional

Table 16. Relation of maternal death rate to age and antenatal care,
Eastern Nigeria[a]

Maternal age (years)	Maternal death rate (per thousand)		Total
	Antenatal care	No antenatal care	
< 14	5	42	27
15	0	58	31
16	0	18	8
17–19	1	21	7
20–24	1	14	4
25–29	1	18	5
≥ 30	2	28	11
all ages	1	24	8
Total no. of maternal deaths	13	161	174
Total no. of mothers	14 396	6 693	21 089

[a] Reproduced, by permission, from: HARRISON, K.A. & ROSSITER, C.E. Zaria (Nigeria) maternity survey 1976–1979. III. The influence of maternal age and parity on childbearing with special reference to primigravidae aged 15 years and under. *British journal of obstetrics and gynaecology* (in press).

Table 17. Infant mortality (per 1000 live births) by age of mother at time of birth[a]

Country or territory	Maternal age (years)		
	< 20	20–29	30–39
Bangladesh	174.3	113.5	113.0
Indonesia	125.2	88.1	88.6
Jamaica	38.5	34.6	56.6
Malaysia	57.9	37.0	35.8
Mexico	86.8	67.2	79.8
Sri Lanka	71.8	57.3	55.3
Thailand	102.0	66.8	74.7

[a] Reproduced, by permission, from: RUTSTEIN, S.O. *Infant and child mortality. Levels, trends and demographic differentials.* London, World Fertility Survey, 1983 (Comparative Studies, Cross-national Summaries, No. 24).

requirements not only for the growth of the fetus but also for the mother herself, and, if they are not met, her future physical health may be impaired (57).

However, to examine only the biological aspects of pregnancy in adolescence is to take too narrow an approach, for the psychological and social consequences are of equal importance. In some traditional societies, such pregnancy is an integral part of the culture and occurs under the protection of the family and society. While the medical risks for the younger adolescent remain, the emotional consequences are likely to be very different from those created when pregnancy occurs unexpectedly to a frightened teenager who

Table 18. Causes of perinatal mortality in England and Wales, 1979[a]

Cause	Perinatal mortality per 1000 total births		Relative risk
	Maternal age < 20 years	Maternal age ≥ 20 years	
Congenital malformation	3.8	3.1	1.2
Complication of placenta cord and prematurity	6.2	4.3	1.4
Hypoxia and other respiratory conditions	4.6	2.8	1.6
Difficult labour and birth injury	0.6	0.5	1.1
Maternal condition	1.6	1.4	1.1
Miscellaneous	3.0	2.0	1.5
All causes	19.7	14.1	1.4

[a] Reproduced, by permission, from: VISUVANATHAN, S. & EDOUARD, L. Trends in adolescent pregnancy. *Journal of obstetrics and gynaecology* (in press).

anticipates serious social disapproval when her condition becomes known. In the latter instance, a pregnancy is often kept secret as long as possible, with the result that antenatal care is likely to be delayed or non-existent or induced abortion is resorted to late in gestation, increasing the risk to health. The younger and more disadvantaged, who are in need of proper nutrition, psychological support, and economic help, are least likely to obtain help because of their lack of experience and resources. If they are schoolchildren, their education is likely to come to an abrupt halt, together with the opportunity for further training. If they are employed, they are likely to lose their jobs unless there is protective legislation. If they are unemployed, they lose the possibility of achieving economic independence and may become even more impoverished, to the detriment of their own health and that of the baby, if it is born. A sense of shame, guilt, or inadequacy may grow and further damage the young woman who becomes pregnant. In many cases having a baby means isolation from peer groups and the loss of social learning experience at a crucial time. Marriage as a consequence of the pregnancy may also mean an involvement in adult and parental responsibilities for which the young couple is neither prepared nor sufficiently mature (1). Adolescents with children may also require more support from their parents, who may not be able or willing to provide it. As a result, their existing social instability is aggravated —a situation that may lead to divorce, with further adverse psychosocial consequences.

A teenage couple or a teenage mother cannot be expected to have reached the necessary level of maturity for rearing a child and providing it with the physical and mental stimulation needed for optimum growth and development. This may lead to an increased incidence of childhood illnesses and disturbances with a "battered child" as a consequence (*58, 59*). In the most serious cases, children may be abandoned or victims of infanticide.

There is clear evidence that adolescents in developed countries are liable to resort to abortion as a way out of unwanted pregnancies or forced marriage (Table 19). Even where therapeutic abortion is

Table 19. Legal abortions per 100 known pregnancies for women under 20 years of age[a]

Country or territory	Year	Age of women		
		≤ 14 years	15–17 years	18–19 years
Canada	1980	46.5	38.2	27.5
Czechoslovakia	1980	24.5	19.7	12.4
England and Wales[b]	1979	60.6	38.4	23.2
German Democratic Republic	1975	33.1	23.6	15.9
Hungary	1979	23.1	26.3	21.6
New Zealand	1979	23.2	16.1	7.9
Norway	1979	85.7	53.7	30.3
Sweden	1979	87.8	63.0	37.1
USA	1980	41.7	41.7	39.6

[a] Reproduced, by permission, from: TIETZE, C. *Induced abortions: a world review, 1983.* New York, The Population Council, 1983, p. 51.
[b] Residents only.

available, it is frequently too late for a simple one-time intervention such as vacuum aspiration or dilatation and curettage, with the result that more complicated procedures such as two-step abortions or hysterotomies are called for. This increases physical and psychological stress. The risks are even more obvious when social and legal circumstances predispose the girl concerned to resort to an unlicensed practitioner.

In an increasing number of countries, legislation on abortion has been liberalized, and it is often available on request to women during the first trimester of pregnancy. But, even where it is culturally acceptable, it is not so simple for a young girl without support, resources, or social preparedness to seek an abortion early enough. Perhaps the most important point that needs to be made about the problems associated with teenage pregnancy is that they can be

prevented by ensuring that there are fewer high-risk mothers (*60*).
Table 16 suggests that antenatal care may do a great deal to reduce
mortality among young mothers.

4.6.3 *Sexually transmitted disease*

More than 20 disease agents are now known to be transmitted
sexually. The full extent of the problem is difficult to determine
because of universal underreporting. Also, national statistics are
often collected in different ways and do not lend themselves to
comparison. Some recent data from the USA (Table 20) show that

Table 20. Trends in annual incidence of sexually transmitted diseases
(per 100 000 population), by age, USA, 1956–1982[a]

Year	Primary and secondary syphilis		Gonorrhoea	
	15–19 years	20–24 years	15–19 years	20–24 years
1956	10.7	18.4	415.7	781.8
1960	19.8	45.9	412.7	859.2
1977	13.8	30.4	1214.8	2013.5
1978	14.6	30.8	1228.9	1977.6
1979	16.2	35.3	1211.4	1780.5
1980	16.9	35.8	1168.3	1775.8
1981	20.7	41.7	1208.8	1775.8
1982	23.1	44.9	1200.2	1724.2

[a] From information available to WHO.

adolescents aged 15–19 years and young adults from 20–24 years
bear a disproportionate share of the increase in reported cases of
syphilis and gonorrhoea. In developed countries, more than two-
thirds of all reported cases of gonorrhoea occur among persons
under 25 years.

The continuing high incidence of salpingitis among young females
bodes ill for the future. Pelvic inflammatory disease not only involves
short-term risks but can also lead to serious complications, including
ectopic pregnancy, tubo-ovarian abscess, and infertility. It has been
estimated that 12–20% of females with untreated gonorrhoea will
eventually develop salpingitis. Moreover, because of unique
biological characteristics and/or sexual and social behaviour, young
females may be even more susceptible than older females to the
increasingly frequent gonococcal and chlamydial infections. Fig. 9
shows that, for acute pelvic inflammatory disease, there is a sharp
peak in hospitalization rates at ages 20–24 years.

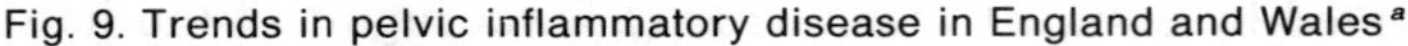

Fig. 9. Trends in pelvic inflammatory disease in England and Wales[a]

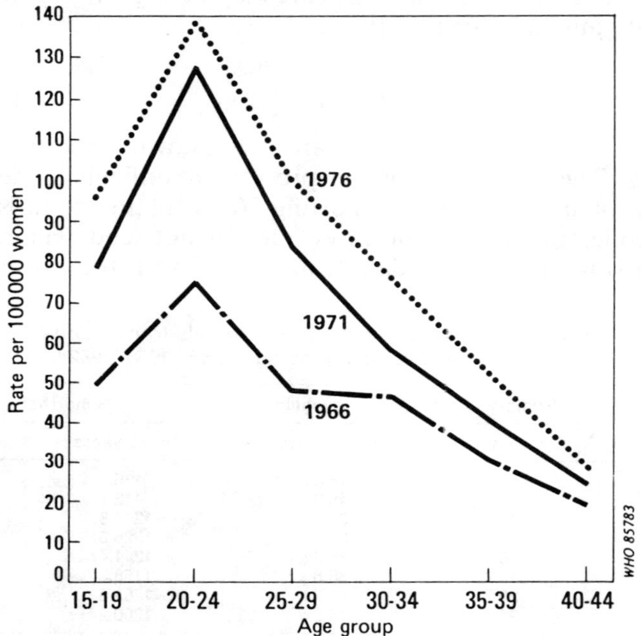

[a] Source: ROBINSON, N., ET AL. Trends in pelvic inflammatory disease in England and Wales. *Journal of epidemiology and community health*, **35**: 265–270 (1981).

The scanty information available on sexually transmitted disease among adolescents in developing countries comes from *ad hoc* surveys. Such data as exist indicate infection rates that are at least as high as those observed in developed countries. Even more seriously, the scarcity of adequate diagnostic and curative services makes it likely that the vast majority of infections will go untreated, so that problems of infertility and ectopic pregnancies may be expected later on.

4.6.4 *Sexual abuse in adolescence*

A useful definition of sexual abuse is "the involvement of dependent, developmentally immature children and adolescents in sexual activities that they do not comprehend, to which they are unable to give informed consent, or that violate the social taboo of family roles" (*61*).

Over the past ten years, there has been increasing evidence of sexual exploitation of children and adolescents (especially females) within families. There also appears to be an alarming increase in rape. Programmes dealing with family problems are needed to a greater extent than before and those that already exist should be specially prepared to deal with relationships between adolescents and their families. Crisis intervention programmes are needed to deal with the aftermath of rape.

4.6.5 *Prostitution of adolescents*

This phenomenon, which involves males as well as females, appears to be increasing in both developed and developing countries. It is a highly complex issue often linked with familial and socioeconomic problems, and sometimes with alcohol and drug abuse. In developing countries, it is associated with the increase in tourism and the migration of young people from relatively structured rural environments to an unprotected life in industrialized urban areas. Prostitution in adolescence, apart from being degrading in itself, brings with it many health problems including unwanted pregnancy, sexually transmitted disease, and emotional disturbance. There is a growing need for measures to prevent its spread, and for the rehabilitation of youthful prostitutes. These can only be effective as part of a broader health and social welfare programme that takes into account the alternative life-styles available to young people.

4.7 Biological and medical problems

4.7.1 *Common medical problems of adolescence*

The surge in sex steroids during puberty causes the rather dramatic changes in anthropometry and body composition commonly referred to as "the adolescent growth spurt". The development of adolescents is particularly vulnerable to adverse influences such as inadequate nutrition, infections, and social and economic privation.

The normal changes of puberty hold great personal significance for adolescents. A heightened awareness of bodily change is normal, and real or imaginary problems relating to development or health can cause anxiety and distress. Girls may be particularly sensitive about unequal breast size, although greater symmetry generally occurs with time. Between 19% and 64% of boys develop mild gynaecomastia around mid-puberty (*62*) but this generally subsides spontaneously in 6–18 months. Occasionally it is more marked and persistent, causing acute psychological distress, and surgical excision may be required.

For adolescents who are developmentally out of step with their peers, the psychological effects can be great. Delayed puberty, with or without short stature, is most commonly due to constitutional factors, but other causes such as chronic disease or endocrine dysfunction must not be excluded. Excessive tallness, which may be particularly difficult for girls, is usually genetic, one or both parents being tall. Whether the problem be shortness or tallness, accurate assessment is important, counselling and objective reassurance essential, and hormonal intervention sometimes justified.

Menstrual disorders are common in adolescence during the period when endocrine maturation is occurring. The commonest abnormality is secondary amenorrhoea, while primary amenorrhoea is rare. Menarche is delayed by undernutrition and strenuous physical exercise. Oligomenorrhoea (infrequent menses) is common during the first few years after menarche and does not require an intervention, such as hormonal regulation, unless it is persistent or severe. However, girls with a history of cycles over two months long for more than two years are likely to suffer from persistent menstrual problems and infertility due to defective ovaluation (*63*). Repeated heavy menstrual bleeding is rare and also associated with relatively poor reproductive potential. Dysmenorrhoea is very common in adolescence and can occasionally be severe and disabling.

Acne is universal in adolescence, with no young person escaping a few comedones and pustules and about 80% having manifest disease. Other skin conditions occurring frequently in young people include warts, atopic eczema, tinea cruris, and scabies. During early adolescence, a number of orthopaedic conditions are found that rarely occur in other age groups. Idiopathic scoliosis occurs predominantly in girls, whilst Osgood-Schlatter disease and slipped upper femoral epiphysis are more commen in boys.

Throughout the world, there is a paucity of data on the incidence and prevalence of medical problems in adolescence. In developing countries where the majority of adolescents live in rural areas, infections of the respiratory and gastrointestinal systems are particularly common. A very high prevalence of dental caries has been observed among the adolescent populations of a number of developing countries. Dental hygiene, reparative services, and preventive measures such as fluoridation are limited or non-existent in many areas.

4.7.2 *Nutrition-related disorders*

The problems of under- and overnutrition in adolescence and youth are important. Normally, as a result of increases in growth rate and physical activity, adolescents have relatively high nutritional requirements. In particular, the energy demands of puberty are high, and the timing of the growth spurt is of major relevance. Boys double their body weight between 10 and 16 years of age (*64*). Pregnancy and intensive training for sport also increase nutritional needs (*65*).

(*a*) *Malnutrition.* In developing countries, 20–30% of children suffer from malnutrition (*66*). While this mainly affects preschool children, lost ground cannot be made up. Many young children with mild to moderate malnutrition survive to reach adolescence, when the malnutrition tends to remain mild but chronic, being detectable only by anthropometric measurements. On the other hand, relatively well-nourished children may develop protein-energy malnutrition in adolescence as a result of acquired dietary habits.

Two types of malnutrition can be recognized in young people: (i) circumstantial and (ii) preferential. The former is due to lack of food; the latter a consequence of self-imposed diets.

(i) Poverty is the most important cause of malnutrition in all age groups in developing countries. In India, for example, where nearly half the country's population lives below the poverty level, the incidence of undernutrition in young people is likely to be high (*67*). Families lacking the financial resources to buy food are frequently large, which compounds the problem. Malnutrition lowers resistance to infections, which themselves exaggerate features of malnutrition (the immunological basis for this has been extensively studied (*68*)). Malnutrition constitutes a particular risk factor for pregnancy in adolescence and is a well-recognized cause of low birth weight in developing countries.

(ii) Preferential malnutrition is of relevance in both developing and developed countries. In the former, in areas where nutritious food is available, it may not be consumed because of certain beliefs and taboos. In developed countries in particular "food faddism" and extreme diets can lead to nutritional imbalance or physical illness, despite relative affluence. An obsession with thinness as the ideal body form is significantly related to media stereotypes.

So-called "fast-food" is making its presence felt throughout the world. It should be noted that, in general terms, if energy intake is adequate, other nutrients will be satisfactory (with the exception of iron in females). In healthy adolescents, homeostatic mechanisms can be trusted to ensure adequate energy intake, and it is now accepted that snacks contribute to a well-rounded diet. However, most fast-food is excessively high in fat and salt.

(b) Obesity. Owing to the normal increased distribution of body fat prior to and during puberty, some adolescents are vulnerable to excessive weight gain at this time. Others have been overweight since childhood as a result of predominantly constitutional factors or overfeeding, although, in rare instances, endocrine causes or unusual syndromes are involved. The precise role of hypercellularity of the adipose tissue organ in the genesis of juvenile obesity remains controversial and unclear. There are also psychodynamic factors of significance in understanding and dealing with this problem (*69*).

A variety of methods exists for identifying obesity in young people, although, in practice, if they look fat, they usually are fat. A greater challenge is treatment which, in the case of adolescents, has been less than satisfactory. The important issue is that teenagers are normally in a state of anabolism during their period of growth. The treatment of obesity by reducing energy intake results in catabolism, the complete antithesis of anabolism, and, if prolonged, may interfere with growth. It should also be remembered that demanding a change of life-style is likely to be unrealistic and stress-inducing during adolescence. Current thinking on this subject favours modest short-term goals, such as maintaining weight while the growth spurt proceeds, and support in the form of supervised peer group activities.

The risk of cardiovascular and other conditions in later life is, however, of special concern, and there is a need for further research into the etiology of these conditions and ways of forestalling them.

4.8 Chronic and disabling conditions

It is estimated that about 10% of the world's population is disabled. The incidence of disability in adolescence is considered to be within the range of 5–8%. In the year 2000 the number of adolescents is expected to be 1180 million; this would mean, at the lowest estimate, a population of 59 million disabled adolescents at the end of the millenium.

Since each disabled adolescent is in close contact with at least three other persons—in the family or in the community—this would mean at least an additional 177 million persons whose lives would be closely affected by the incidence of disabilities in adolescents. These figures are staggering in their implications, especially for the future of disabled adolescents in the developing countries where population growth is most rapid.

Many young people have been disabled from birth or childhood. Medical progress and rigorous management have enabled increasing numbers of them to reach adolescence. Once there, they constitute a particularly vulnerable group in whom many aspects of growth and development are adversely affected. In developing countries, where basic needs have priority and, in particular, where access to medical and supportive care is limited, children with diseases and handicaps are less likely to survive.

The importance of accidents as a cause of injury in adolescence has already been emphasized. Trauma related to traffic, work, sport, or physical assault is the commonest cause of disabilities acquired in adolescence, since it may result in amputation, spinal injury, or brain injury.

Common chronic and disabling conditions often seen in adolescence are listed below:

Physical handicaps

- dwarfism
- cerebral palsy/paresis
- visual, hearing, or speech defects
- spina bifida/other genetic disorders
- facial deformity
- traumatic lesions
- marked obesity

Intellectual handicaps

- learning disorders
- mental retardation

Chronic disease

- epilepsy
- asthma/cystic fibrosis
- diabetes
- juvenile rheumatoid arthritis
- cardiovascular disorders
- inflammatory bowel disease
- malignancy
- neurological infection

In adolescents, certain disease states may exhibit different characteristics or require a particular approach for their medical management. Epilepsy, for example, may have its onset during adolescence, or there may be an exacerbation of seizure activity. Traditionally, it has been considered inadvisable to withdraw anticonvulsants during puberty. The results of a recent survey dispute this (70). Asthma is often associated with additional problems in teenagers, who may deny symptoms or suffer stress. Diabetes mellitus, perhaps the most important chronic disorder in young people, becomes more difficult to control during periods of rapid growth. It can cause havoc in families that are already vulnerable or dysfunctional (71).

4.8.1 Impact of illness and disability

The process of adolescence is far from being the same for the young person with a chronic illness or disability as it is for his or her healthy peers. There are many obstacles to the achievement of important developmental tasks and a variety of behavioural responses that often exacerbate the difficulties.

—Enforced dependency and continuing overprotectiveness by parents may interfere with efforts to separate from the family. Many disabled young people go through periods of denial, anger, and demands for compensation from parents and/or society. Noncompliance with medical and rehabilitation regimens often represents an effort to achieve a measure of self-determination and should be viewed in a developmental and situational context.
—As sensitivity about body image is greatest during adolescence, and as the process of establishing a psychosexual identity depends initially on acceptance of one's own body, any deformity or imperfection, obvious or hidden, can have an adverse affect. Sometimes, and with certain disabilities, reactions may reach the level of considering one's body and its defects with disgust, shame, and loathing. Acceptance of one's own sexuality also presents problems, and opportunities for sexual expression are limited.
—Interference with educational or vocational goals by illness or injury creates anxiety about the prospect of future economic independence. Other obstacles to independence include

bureaucratic and organizational factors as well as prejudices in the labour market.

—Social isolation results from problems of mobility, transport, and access, shyness and poor self-esteem, lack of social skills, and difficulties with bodily functions, combined with lack of acceptance by peers who are not disabled. Loneliness is often the greatest handicap of all for the disabled adolescent, impairing the development of a positive adult self-identity.

The intrinsic problems facing chronically ill and disabled young people are greatly compounded by certain attitudes and behaviour. The concept of "spread of disability" (*72*) is based on: the tendency of people (parents, professionals, the general public, and the disabled themselves) to view a disabled person through the "keyhole" of the disability, rather than as a *person* with a disability (e.g., as an "epileptic" rather than a person with epilepsy); the prevalence of a variety of labels, stereotypes, and mythical concepts (e.g., retarded persons are sexually aggressive); unrealistically low expectations; the ascription of certain types of "normal" and developmentally based behaviour (e.g., moodiness, insecurity, rebelliousness) to the disability; other forms of stigmatization (e.g., viewing a disabled person as inferior, as something odd, or as a threat to one's conscience or emotional comfort).

4.9 Occupational health problems

From the beginning of the Industrial Revolution, children and young people have worked in factories and mines. Although it is illegal in most countries to employ child labour, it was estimated that in 1983, 50 million children under the age of 15 were at work (*73*), the vast majority in developing countries. Most of these children had no opportunity to go to school and were forced to work because of economic conditions. Child labour is an indicator of poverty and underdevelopment; most working children are employed in agriculture or small-scale industries.

4.9.1 *Health problems at the place of work*

Young people are particularly vulnerable to certain problems and diseases that can be ameliorated by the use of ergonomics, a science in which machines are looked upon as extension of human sensory and locomotive activity. Mechanical devices made with a view to accommodating the physical dimensions of the operator are satisfactory from the ergonomic standpoint. Children should not be permitted to work with machines or equipment made for adults since this practice leads to premature fatigue, accidents, and injuries (*74*). Children who have to work in very confined areas or in awkward positions may develop physical deformities, backache, or arthritis.

Young people are also at greater risk in their occupational environment because of their lack of experience. The occupational environment contains a variety of chemical, physical, and biological hazards. For example, exposure to certain dusts can lead to chronic lung disease. Young people may not have information or knowledge about these hazards and sometimes, even if they have the information, they may not be willing or able to take the necessary steps to protect themselves.

5. LEGAL AND POLICY ASPECTS OF HEALTH CARE FOR YOUNG PEOPLE

5.1 Laws and policies affecting health services for young people

Law and policy[1] have an important influence on health programmes for young people. They may be supportive of health care in some areas and not in others. The definition of "youth" in law and policy varies. In law, one becomes an adult at the age of "majority" which may differ from place to place. The designated age of adulthood is important because it is the age at which young people can individually exercise free choice by giving consent. In the health care system, consent is the key to access. Until recently, an almost universal rule has been that "minors", as they are termed in law, must have the consent of their parents or some other adult, before they can obtain health care and advice. This has tended to inhibit young people from seeking health care where sensitive issues are involved, and medical and health care personnel from providing it.

In this area, the critical issue is: at what age, or, better still, at what stage of individual development, should a young person be able

---

[1] The term "law and policy", as used here, comprises: legislation, judicial decisions, ministerial norms and policy statements, administrative regulations, executive decrees, attorney general's opinions, codes of professional associations, and, in some instances, constitutional, customary, and religious law, as well as professional practice. All of these create legal and policy norms that may impinge on health care programmes.

to take decisions on his or her health care? Where there is an age restriction, what should the providers of health care do when somebody under age seeks out such care, but does not want parental involvement? Some countries have addressed the issue by lowering the age of majority for purposes of medical treatment; some have enacted a "health services to minors act" that permits people who are under age to seek and consent to health care in specific areas, i.e., veneral disease, drug abuse, sexual problems, and pregnancy; others have moved toward the use of the "emancipated minor" rule, which recognizes that adolescents who are independent financially and in such matters as life-style should be capable of giving consent.

Legally, consent given must be "informed", which means that the consenting person must understand:

—the nature of the medical procedure to be used;
—the risks and seriousness of the suggested procedure;
—the potential benefits;
—the need for any post-treatment supervision or continued treatment;
—the alternatives to the treatment suggested and the relative risks and benefits involved; and
—the right to refuse treatment and the consequences of doing so, as well as the assurance that no punitive action will result from a refusal.

In any case, to ensure adequate understanding by young people, counselling as well as information may be needed.

5.1.1 *Mental health*

In 1955, WHO reported (*75*) that the mental health laws of many countries, often carried over from the nineteenth century, did not always reflect current thought and did not provide a good basis for the development of progressive programmes in mental health. Since 1955, major changes have occurred regarding techniques of treatment, the organization of mental health care, and the protection of human rights. There has been a move towards voluntary hospitalization, more flexible legal admission and discharge policies, and an encouragement of greater interaction between patient, family, and professional staff. The emphasis has been away from mainly custodial care towards less centralized types of service, including crisis intervention and day, foster, and community care.

The extent to which adolescents have access to these facilities varies from country to country.

Austria, France, and Scotland furnish examples of community-based preventive programmes and crisis intervention centres located within the general hospital framework. The access of young people to these services is socially accepted. Sweden, as well, has developed services with separate psychiatric units for young people up to 18 years of age on a district basis, making the field of mental health care not so much a specialized branch of medicine as a public health concern.

However, most countries have yet to move significantly toward community-based mental health care and, in some countries where major changes have occurred, the existing laws clash with current programme objectives (76). The lag between legislation, innovative mental health programmes, and the availability of mental health care geared to the needs of all groups of society (including adolescents) is great. A critical review of existing mental health legislation is desirable with a view to setting up the framework to meet these needs.

5.1.2 *Sexual and reproductive health*

Legislation on sexual and reproductive health in adolescence is still a controversial area, involving sensitive issues such as sex education, information and counselling, pregnancy prevention, abortion, and sexually transmitted diseases. It is estimated that 75% of adolescents under 15 years of age (and 50% of those over 15) throughout the world, have no access to programmes of information and education on reproductive health. This must be considered an undesirable situation, putting vast numbers of sexually active young people at risk. Beyond knowing the mechanics of sex, young people need a greater understanding of the role of sex in the realm of human relationships.

With regard to law and policy on formal sex education, the following are key questions.

—Should courses on reproductive health be permitted within the school curriculum?
—If so, should these courses be obligatory or elective?
—What should the content of the courses be?
—Should they be separate or integrated into other, ongoing courses?

—Should they be given separately to each sex or not? Does this depend on age?

—What role should parents have? Is their consent required? To what extent should they be allowed to screen the material used in courses?

Basically, there are five different types of legal response to these questions: (1) to make sex education compulsory; (2) to make it elective; (3) to approve of sex education but without legislation on the matter; (4) neither to prohibit sex education nor to promote it; and (5) to prohibit some aspects of sex education completely or partially.

While sex education programmes in a formal setting constitute one of the best ways of reaching a broad adolescent audience, it is also true that, throughout the world, a large number of those who need to be reached do not have the chance of formal education.[1] Other ways of reaching them must be sought, but the laws regarding the public dissemination of information on sexual health are often restrictive.

Contraception is, in the opinion of many, the keystone of any rational approach to the problem of the sexually active adolescent. It is here that law and policy are important. The law determines who has access to contraception and under what conditions. Where contraception is acceptable for adolescents, it is not always available to those who are unmarried (see Table 21).

Legislation concerning induced abortion varies widely throughout the world (Table 22). Experience has clearly shown that women in need will turn to abortion as a method of coping with unwanted pregnancies, whether it is legal or not. Adolescents seem to be no different and, indeed, are much more vulnerable than adults to the risks associated with abortion. In 1983, 30% of all abortions in the USA were performed on women under 20 years of age. The

---

[1] School populations are very large in Europe and North America, with nearly all young people attending school until they are 16 or 17. However, in many developing countries, the situation is rather different. School-leaving ages are much lower—often between 12 and 14. In some countries, there are no schools for children to attend in many rural areas. Data published by the World Bank show that more than 50% of European children of secondary-school age attend school. However, the corresponding rates elsewhere are: only 36% in Latin America, 22% in North Africa and the Middle East, 20% in Southern Asia, and 6.9% in Africa (south of the Sahara). WORLD BANK. *World Bank economic indicators.* Washington, DC, World Bank, 1979 (Report No. 700/79/01).

Table 21. Laws and policies on availability of contraceptives (certain countries)

Country or territory	Type of contraceptive				Comments
	Condom	Pill	IUD	Other	
Brazil	A	A P		A	Health Ministry supplies contraceptives to needy persons under 20 years of age (high-risk group); IUDs prohibited (1977)
France	A	A P	A P	A	under-age unmarried persons may get contraceptives at family centres (1974)
Gabon	A P	A P	A P	A P	contraceptives supplied for therapeutic reasons only, on advice of three doctors; even then they are available to those under 25 years of age only if "absolutely" necessary (1965)
Hungary	A	A P (16 yrs)	A P (18 yrs)	A	16–18-year-olds must be dealt with by an obstetrician/gynaecologist (1974)
Indonesia	A	A P	A P	A	providing contraceptives to persons under 17 years is technically a crime; contraceptives available to married persons only
Mexico	A	A P	A P	A	contraceptives technically unavailable to young unmarried persons (1974)
New Zealand	A	A P	A P	A P	persons under 16 years of age may get contraceptives at family planning centres (1977)
Papua New Guinea	A	A	A P	A	contraceptives available to young married persons only; consent of spouse required (1979)
Saudi Arabia	–	–	–	–	contraception banned (1975)
Sweden	A	A P	A P	A	doctors forbidden to inform parents
Thailand	A	A P	A P	A	contraception available to all adolescents (1970)

A = Available. P = Prescription required from doctor or auxiliary health worker.

Table 22. Legal status of abortion by country or territory and by grounds, mid-1982 [a]

Country or territory	Illegal [b]	Legal on specified grounds [c]					
		Medical		Eugenic (fetal)	Juridical (rape, incest, etc.)	Social and social-medical	Legal (grounds not specified)
		Narrow (life)	Broad (health)				
Afghanistan	—	×	—	—	—	—	—
Albania	—	—	×	—	—	—	—
Algeria	—	—	×	—	—	—	—
Argentina	—	—	×	—	×	—	—
Australia	—	—	×	× [d]	—	× [e, f]	—
Austria	—	—	—	—	—	—	× [g, h]
Bangladesh	—	×	—	—	—	—	—
Belgium	—	×	—	—	—	—	—
Benin	—	×	—	—	—	—	—
Bolivia	—	—	×	—	×	—	—
Brazil	—	×	—	—	×	—	—
Bulgaria [i]	—	—	×	×	×	× [j]	—
Burkina Faso	×	—	—	—	—	—	—
Burma	—	×	—	—	—	—	—
Burundi	×	—	—	—	—	—	—
Cameroon	—	—	×	—	×	—	—
Canada	—	—	×	—	—	—	—
Central African Republic	×	—	—	—	—	—	—
Chad	—	×	—	—	—	—	—
Chile	—	×	—	—	—	—	—
China	—	—	—	—	—	—	× [k]
Colombia	—	×	—	—	—	—	—
Congo	—	—	×	—	—	—	—
Costa Rica	—	—	×	—	—	—	—
Ivory Coast	—	×	—	—	—	—	—
Cuba	—	—	—	—	—	—	× [j]
Czechoslovakia	—	—	×	×	×	× [g]	—
Democratic Yemen	—	×	—	—	—	—	—
Democratic People's Republic of Korea [l]	—	—	×	×	×	×	—
Denmark	—	—	—	—	—	—	× [g]
Dominican Republic	×	—	—	—	—	—	—
Ecuador	—	×	—	—	×	—	—
Egypt	×	—	—	×	—	—	—
El Salvador	—	×	—	×	×	—	—
Ethiopia	—	—	×	—	—	—	—
Finland [m]	—	—	×	×	×	× [g]	—
France	—	—	—	—	—	—	× [j]
Germany, Democratic Republic of	—	—	—	—	—	—	× [g]

Table 22 (continued)

Country or territory	Illegal[b]	Legal on specified grounds[c]					
		Medical		Eugenic (fetal)	Juridical (rape, incest, etc.)	Social and social-medical	Legal (grounds not specified)
		Narrow (life)	Broad (health)				
Germany, Federal Republic of	—	—	×	×	×	×[g, h]	—
Ghana	—	—	×	—	—	—	—
Greece	—	—	×	×	—	—	—
Guatemala	—	×	—	—	—	—	—
Guinea	—	—	×	—	—	—	—
Haiti	×	—	—	—	—	—	—
Honduras	—	—	×	—	—	—	—
Hong Kong	—	—	×	×	×	—	—
Hungary[n]	—	—	×	×	×	×[g]	—
Iceland	—	—	×	×	×	×[g]	—
India	—	—	×	×	×	×[o]	—
Indonesia	×	—	—	—	—	—	—
Iran, Islamic Republic of	×	—	—	—	—	—	—
Iraq	—	×	—	—	—	—	—
Ireland	—	×	—	—	—	—	—
Israel	—	—	×	×	×	—	—
Italy	—	—	—	—	—	—	×[g]
Jamaica	—	—	×	—	—	—	—
Japan[p]	—	—	×	×	×	×[q]	—
Jordan	—	—	×	—	×	—	—
Kenya	—	—	×	—	—	—	—
Kuwait	—	×	—	—	—	—	—
Laos	—	×	—	—	—	—	—
Lebanon	—	×	—	—	—	—	—
Lesotho	—	×	—	—	—	—	—
Liberia	—	—	×	×	×	—	—
Libyan Arab Jamahiriya	—	×	—	—	—	—	—
Luxembourg	—	—	×	×	×	×[g]	—
Madagascar	—	×	—	—	—	—	—
Malawi	—	×	—	—	—	—	—
Malaysia	—	×	—	×	×	—	—
Mali	×	—	—	—	—	—	—
Malta	×	—	—	—	—	—	—
Mauritania	×	—	—	—	—	—	—
Mexico	—	×	—	—	×	—	—
Mongolia	×	—	—	—	—	—	—
Morocco	—	—	×	—	—	—	—
Mozambique	—	×	—	—	—	—	—

Table 22 *(continued)*

Country or territory	Illegal [b]	Legal on specified grounds [c]					Legal (grounds not specified)
		Medical		Eugenic (fetal)	Juridical (rape, incest, etc.)	Social and social-medical	
		Narrow (life)	Broad (health)				
Namibia	—	—	×	×	×	—	—
Nepal	—	—	×	—	—	—	—
Netherlands	—	—	—	—	—	—	× [f]
New Zealand	—	—	×	×	×	—	—
Nicaragua	—	×	—	—	—	—	—
Niger	×	—	—	—	—	—	—
Nigeria	—	×	—	—	—	—	—
Norway	—	—	—	—	—	—	× [g]
Pakistan	—	×	—	—	—	—	—
Panama	×	—	—	—	—	—	—
Papua New Guinea	—	—	×	—	—	—	—
Paraguay	—	×	—	—	—	—	—
Peru	—	—	×	—	—	—	—
Philippines	×	—	—	—	—	—	—
Poland [p]	—	—	×	—	×	× [g]	—
Portugal	×	—	—	—	—	—	—
Puerto Rico	—	—	—	—	—	—	× [f]
Republic of Korea	—	—	×	×	×	—	—
Romania	—	—	×	×	×	× [g, r]	—
Rwanda	×	—	—	—	—	—	—
Saudi Arabia	—	×	—	—	—	—	—
Senegal	—	×	—	—	—	—	—
Sierra Leone	—	—	×	—	—	—	—
Singapore	—	—	—	—	—	—	× [q]
Somalia	×	—	—	—	—	—	—
South Africa	—	—	×	×	×	—	—
Spain	×	—	—	—	—	—	—
Sri Lanka	—	×	—	—	—	—	—
Sudan	—	×	—	—	—	—	—
Sweden	—	—	—	—	—	—	× [s]
Switzerland	—	—	×	—	—	—	—
Syria	—	×	—	—	—	—	—
Thailand	—	—	×	—	×	—	—
Togo	—	×	—	—	—	—	—
Trinidad & Tobago	—	—	×	—	—	—	—
Tunisia	—	—	—	—	—	—	× [g]
Turkey	—	×	—	×	×	—	—
Uganda	—	—	×	—	—	—	—
United Kingdom [t] England, Scotland, and Wales	—	—	×	×	—	× [f]	—
Northern Ireland	—	×	—	—	—	—	—

Table 22 *(continued)*

Country or territory	Illegal[b]	Legal on specified grounds[c]					
		Medical		Eugenic (fetal)	Juridical (rape, incest, etc.)	Social and social-medical	Legal (grounds not specified)
		Narrow (life)	Broad (health)				
United States of America	—	—	—	—	—	—	× [f]
United Republic of Tanzania	—	—	×	—	—	—	—
Uruguay	—	×	—	—	×	× [u]	—
USSR	—	—	—	—	—	—	× [g]
Venezuela	—	×	—	—	—	—	—
Viet Nam	—	—	—	—	—	—	× [v]
Yemen	—	×	—	—	—	—	—
Yugoslavia	—	—	—	—	—	—	× [j]
Zaire	×	—	—	—	—	—	—
Zambia	—	—	×	×	—	× [f]	—
Zimbabwe	—	—	×	×	×	—	—

[a] Adapted from: TIETZE, C. *Induced abortion. A world review,* 5th ed. New York, The Population Council, 1983.

The table does not include most countries or territories with fewer than one million inhabitants and those for which information on the legal status of abortion was not available. Countries listed in sources as applying Islamic Law appear under "Medical/narrow (life)."

[b] Abortion to save a woman's life may be authorized under general principles of criminal law (state of necessity).

[c] Abortion on medical and eugenic grounds is generally permitted prior to viability of fetus. Abortion on juridical grounds is generally permitted up to the same gestational period as abortion on social or social-medical grounds.

[d] In Northern Territory and South Australia.

[e] In South Australia by legislation, in New South Wales and Victoria by judicial decision.

[f] Prior to viability of fetus.

[g] During first 3 months or 12 weeks of gestation.

[h] From implantation.

[i] On request for unmarried women, married women with two living children, and married women aged over 40 years with one living child.

[j] During first 10 weeks of gestation.

[k] No legal limit, but most abortions performed during first trimester.

[l] For "important reasons".

[m] On request for women aged over 40 years.

[n] On request for unmarried women, for married women with three living children or those who have experienced three deliveries, for certain categories of women with two living children, for married women aged over 40 years, and for women without a home or apartment of their own.

[o] During first 20 weeks of gestation.

[p] No formal authorization required and abortion permitted in doctor's office; abortion *de facto* available on request.

[q] During first 24 weeks of gestation.

[r] On request for women aged over 40 years and for those with 4 or more living children.

[s] During first 18 weeks of gestation.

[t] The Abortion Act of 1967 does not apply to Northern Ireland.

[u] Penalty may be waived when abortion is performed during first 3 months of pregnancy because of serious economic difficulty.

[v] Gestational limit not ascertained.

figures for some other countries were: England and Wales, 27.3%; Denmark 17.8%; Singapore, 8.8%; India, 6.3%; Czechoslovakia, 6.1%; and Tunisia, 2.5% (*77*). Whether the termination of pregnancy is legally available at all is largely determined by the position taken in the national legislation, and this may vary from a highly restrictive one based on "risk to the life of the woman" (Chile, Iraq, Nigeria, Sri Lanka) to abortion on request, usually during the first trimester (Austria, Singapore, Tunisia, USA) (*78*).

The whole subject of health care for pregnant adolescents must be put in perspective. It is estimated that only 55% of births in the world are attended by trained personnel. Even fewer take place in health institutions (*78a*). In countries where health facilities are available, legislation has tended not to focus on the special needs of adolescents. By and large, services are aimed at all women irrespective of age, though adolescents would seem to be covered by the programmes for "high risk" women in many countries.

The prevention and treatment of sexually transmitted disease (STD) in adolescents is a problem that merits special attention. Most legislation on the subject tends to address all age groups, requiring mandatory treatment and, in some countries, disclosure of the source of infection (if possible) and the names of others who might be affected. (Sometimes secrecy is guaranteed to avoid any social stigma.) In the case of minors, a number of countries have enacted laws or portions of laws expressly authorizing them to have access to treatment. These laws appear to be of three general kinds:

—those enabling minors, irrespective of age, to consent to treatment for sexually transmitted diseases;
—those allowing minors of a certain age to seek out and consent to treatment (these establish a minimum age for treatment); and
—those requiring parental approval before treatment is given.

Because sexually transmitted diseases are reaching epidemic proportions in many parts of the world, there is an urgent need for legislation to facilitate their early detection and treatment by enabling minors to have easy, confidential, and free access to the appropriate services.

5.1.3 *Smoking*

As far as minors are concerned, cigarette smoking has been subjected to relatively little legislation. Though it is the oldest form of anti-smoking legislation, still only a few countries have made it illegal to sell cigarettes to anyone under 16 years of age. However, legislation restricting or prohibiting advertisements that directly or indirectly promote smoking has been increasingly common in recent years. Vigorous anti-smoking campaigns exist, however, and have been successful in some countries, for example Norway and Sweden.

Among the measures suggested are: (*a*) prohibition of the sale of tobacco products to minors; (*b*) restrictions on the sale of cigarettes from automatic vending machines; (*c*) prohibition of smoking in schools and other places frequented by young people; (*d*) prohibition of all smoking in public; (*e*) prohibition of cigarette advertising at times, and in places and ways, calculated to ensure its maximum impact on adolescents (see Table 23); (*f*) establishment of mandatory public health education on the health consequences of smoking; and (*g*) insistence on the placing of mandatory health warnings on cigarette packages.

5.1.4 *Alcohol and drug abuse*

In an increasing number of countries, the uncontrolled use of alcohol and other non-prescription drugs by young people has reached near-epidemic proportions. Drinking by adults, who serve as role models for the young, is legally and socially acceptable in most countries. The minimum age at which minors may legally have access to alcoholic beverages has, in recent years, been raised in some countries (see Table 24). There is also legislation controlling the distribution of alcohol. In some places, there are restrictions on advertisements, aimed at the young, that glamorize the use of alcohol and tobacco. Experience suggests that (*a*) "the area surrounding legal control of alcoholic beverages and consumption is a controversial one and should be approached cautiously and thoughtfully", and (*b*) "a series of restrictions, established after careful consideration of local socio-cultural and economic factors, and imposed after widespread public education and discussion and investigation of public attitudes, is likely to result in measurable improvement" (*43*).

5.1.5 *Accidents and high-risk activities*

Accidents constitute one of the main causes of death among adolescents throughout the world. Because of this, and because most

Table 23. Legislation to control tobacco advertising specifically aimed at children and adolescents (certain countries)[a]

Country or territory	Ban on adolescent-oriented advertising	Ban on advertising in selected media	Ban at places frequented by youth	Comments
Belgium		children's periodicals		voluntary agreement with industry not to aim advertising at the young
Ecuador	×	radio, TV	×	no advertisements on television prior to 19h30
France		publications intended for young		ban on sponsorship of youth events by tobacco companies
Germany, Federal Republic of	×			no advertisements on television prior to 19h00
Malaysia		radio, TV		no advertisements before 19h00
Peru		radio, TV		no advertisements before 20h00; no advertisements before 19h00 in places of entertainment attended by minors
Spain	×	radio, TV		no advertisements on programmes intended for the young; none before 21h30; ban on use of adolescents in advertisements
Sweden		newspapers, periodicals		
Switzerland	×		×	
Venezuela		radio, TV		

[a] Based on WAKE, R. ET AL. *A manual on smoking and children.* Geneva, International Union Against Cancer, 1982, pp. 118–120.

accidents are preventable, many of them being the result of human error combined with an environmental hazard, they are an important consideration in any assessment of young people's health.

One estimate of the magnitude of the problem, made by the WHO Regional Office for Europe, suggests that, for every child or adolescent who dies as a result of an accident, another will be permanently handicapped, 10 others will have to be hospitalized for

Table 24. Minimum age (years) for purchase and consumption
of alcoholic beverages (certain countries) [a]

Country or territory	Purchase to carry away	Consumption on premises	Admission to licenced premises
Australia	18	18	
Brazil		18	
France	14 (fermented drinks) 16 (spirits)	14–16 (may consume fermented drinks, if accompanied by adult) 16–18 (may consume fermented drinks) 18 (spirits)	16 (unless accompanied by adult in charge aged over 18)
Germany, Federal Republic of	16	16 (beer, wine) 18 (spirits)	16 (unless accompanied by adult; some other exceptions)
Iceland	21		
India		no consumption by minors in some states; permitted at 18 or 21 in others	
Indonesia		16	
Japan	20	20	18
Mexico	18	18	18
Philippines	21		
Yugoslavia		15	

[a] Reproduced, by permission, from: MOSER, J. *Prevention of alcohol-related problems: an international review of preventive measures, policies and programmes.* Toronto, Alcoholism and Drug Addiction Research Foundation, 1980, pp. 119–121.

approximately 30 days because of injuries, and about 1000 will suffer an accident that does not require hospitalization (*79*).

Because motor vehicles play such an important role in accidents, legislation on accident prevention is largely concerned with them. This legislation has many facets: licensing requirements (health, age limits, and aptitude); use of seat belts; protective headgear for users of two-wheeled vehicles; and the prohibition or restriction of drinking and drug-taking by those operating vehicles. Laws raising the "drinking age" and punishing drunken drivers more firmly have been particularly effective in the USA, wherever they have been enforced, in cutting fatal accident rates among young people. In 1983 alone, 40 states toughened their laws on drunken driving, while 8 raised the drinking age.

Experience in Europe has been different. The overall aim of recent legislation has been to make vehicle operation safer. The tendencies, as far as young people are concerned, seem to be to raise the drinking age, to lower the legally tolerated limits of the level of alcohol in the blood, and to stiffen penalties. Even so, fatalities and injuries caused by young drunken drivers continue to exceed tolerable limits.

In developing countries, the accident rates are often extremely high, for a variety of reasons—rapid urbanization, an influx of motor vehicles, poor roads, lack of experience, a mixture of motorized traffic with other types—and legislation on accident prevention lags behind.

5.1.6 *Occupational health and safety*

In the industrialized world, an enormous body of legislation has accumulated on the occupational health and safety of every kind of worker. Going beyond the practice of prohibiting dangerous work for the young, it aims at protecting all workers at the work site. However, there is often no legislation of this kind in newly industrialized societies.

Legislative measures to protect the young include the stipulation of a minimum age for employment and restrictions on the types of employment young people may engage in, as well as the same safety regulations that apply to the rest of the work force. However, barring young people from some kinds of employment is not likely to be effective where there is poverty, unless alternative means of economic support are provided. This needs to be brought to the attention of policy-makers in order to avoid endangering the health and lives of the young.

5.1.7 *Health care for the handicapped*

Better care for disabled children is one of the most important aims of recent legislation concerning disabled persons. Rehabilitation has been increasingly recognized as a *right,* and prevention is an increasing concern. Providing health care for the handicapped adolescent is, however, no simple matter. Legislators are slowly dealing with such issues as the detection, prevention, and treatment of disablement, the rehabilitation of disabled persons, and state-assisted financial support for the care of the handicapped. In some cases, there is comprehensive legislation on the disabled, in which the young are singled out; this is found mainly in the developed countries. The goal of providing health care to the handicapped adolescent will remain, in a practical sense, largely illusory, in the absence of the appropriate legal and policy decisions.

5.1.8 *Dental care*

Dental care, despite its importance to the health of adolescents is rarely the subject of legislation. In some countries, school-based dental hygiene programmes, as well as the practice of fluoridation (an important feature of the campaign to create the proper environment for dental health), are backed by a number of statutes and regulations.

*   *
*

Throughout the world, law and policy have failed to keep pace with the rapidly evolving needs of adolescents over the past few years. While there is no model form of legislation or policy that will work in every situation, there are many alternative approaches that could alleviate the health problems of the young. The challenge is to get law and policy to deal with the issues in a responsible, helpful way and to monitor their impact scientifically.

6. PARTICIPATION OF YOUNG PEOPLE
IN HEALTH CARE

6.1 Health service needs of the young

To promote the health of young people, it is necessary to assess their needs and the resources available to meet them (bearing in mind that these resources include the young themselves), and also to identify the factors that deter them from using the existing services. Appropriate research is essential in order to facilitate, monitor, and evaluate this process (*80*).

The following are among the special problems that affect young people throughout the world in different degrees:

—socioeconomic disadvantages
—malnutrition
—unemployment and underemployment

—migration from rural to urban areas
—unwanted pregnancy, hazardous childbirth, induced abortion, and sexually transmitted diseases
—tobacco, alcohol, and drug abuse
—accidents and risk-taking behaviour
—emotional problems and suicide
—physical and mental handicaps
—occupationally related injuries and ill-health.

Individual factors such as gender and the stage of adolescence reached will interact with societal factors in determining the degree to which a problem is perceived as being sufficiently important to warrant help. But, because mortality and conventional types of morbidity are relatively low among young people, their health care is often not given sufficient priority. Furthermore, some 75% of all young people live in rural areas where health services are scarce. Those who live in urban areas often have special new problems for which an infrastructure of services is unlikely to exist. The situation is aggravated by the tendency of young people not to make enough use of conventional health services, even when they are available. Below are some of the reasons:

—Adolescents are neither children nor adults and generally do not fit well into existing systems of health care. Adolescents striving for independence are made uncomfortable by health personnel more accustomed to dealing with children and their parents. Services in which the majority of clients are adults can be insensitive to adolescents who are inexperienced in dealing both with the problems of adolescence and with health personnel.
—The young people most in need are those least likely to seek help. They include the socially disadvantaged, such as members of ethnic minorities, adolescent migrants, the homeless, and the unemployed. This is particularly unfortunate, as physical and psychosocial morbidity is high in these groups.
—Certain physical, aesthetic, and organizational features of conventional agencies can put young people off. These include: location of services, appearance of the premises, opening hours, bureaucratic procedures (notably on reception), attitudes of staff, and fragmentation of preventive or therapeutic measures. From the standpoint of young people, the credibility accorded to services is often in inverse proportion to the official recognition they enjoy and their visibility.

—Young people require and expect confidentiality and help that is provided with their voluntary consent by someone in whom they can have confidence. The ethical aspects of relationships between adolescents and health personnel need special consideration if they are to receive the best kind of support.

—The attitudes and skills of those providing the services, in particular the ease with which they relate to young people, are thus extremely important. These are a question of aptitude and training.

—Service charges that cannot be met without help from others can also deter young people from seeking care. In most instances, free treatment is the best policy, particularly as it encourages the most disadvantaged and vulnerable groups to make use of the available services.

—The participation of the young people themselves in various health service activities should be considered. Willingness to attend a given service is likely to be enhanced when the consumer is involved in its organization.

—The evaluation of services, particularly from the standpoints of availability, accessibility, and utilization should have high priority. Both objective and subjective methods of evaluation should be incorporated into services for young people at all stages of development.

The challenge inherent in the issues outlined above is clear. Where existing services cater for a wide range of age groups, or focus primarily on age groups other than adolescents, important changes are needed if their effective utilization by young people is to increase. Similar considerations apply in the establishment of services specially geared to adolescents.

6.2 Specific health measures

In Section 4, a number of health problems of importance to young people were reviewed. Specific measures to deal with these problems are outlined below.

6.2.1 *Sexual and reproductive health*

(*a*) *Sex education.* Many problems of reproductive health in adolescence stem from the ignorance, misconceptions, and uncertainties about sex, conception, and contraception that are

90

prevalent among the young. One way to deal with this situation is to provide sex education courses in schools. While the timing and specific content of such courses remain a matter for debate, there is now a wider acceptance of the idea and a growing recognition that sex education is essential to health. The wish to learn is universal among the young and, where sound information is not provided, other, less reliable sources will be used. An adequate education programme for adolescents should include material on the following topics presented in a way that is appropriate to the cultural context:

—physical, emotional, and social development;
—sexual maturation;
—sexual drives and behaviour;
—human reproduction;
—sexuality in the context of relationships;
—sexual preferences;
—fertility regulation;
—sexually transmitted disease.

In addition to professionally trained health educators, good use can be made of youth workers and peer counsellors. Techniques that encourage discussion, such as keeping groups small and, where feasible, using video or film, should be encouraged. Training is essential to ensure that the educators are themselves familiar and comfortable with the topics and issues presented.

In much of the world, young adolescents do not attend school and may be all the more in need of sound information and advice on sexual matters. Every effort should be made to promote out-of-school services offering opportunities for education and counselling at places of work, in youth clubs, in the context of sporting and leisure activities, and in places where unemployed young people may congegrate. To achieve this, innovative techniques are needed. As with all new approaches, means of evaluating their effectiveness should be built in. One such innovation, already operating in Hong Kong and shortly to be started in Korea, is a telephone counselling service that troubled youngsters can turn to when in need of help.

(b) *Counselling*. As noted above, counselling may take a wide variety of forms, and it should be available in such a way as to inspire trust. Counsellors must be trained to be sensitive to the needs and wishes of young people and themselves sufficiently knowledgeable about questions of sex and reproduction either to provide help or to refer inquiries to those who can. They can play a vital role by providing a more objective viewpoint than family or friends, and in some cases, a broader outlook than the actual providers of services. Counselling should be considered an essential feature of reproductive health services for the young (*81*).

(*c*) *Specific services*. For virtually every aspect of sexual behaviour and reproductive health in adolescence, some services are needed. It is important not only that such services should be available but that they should be accessible to all young people, males as well as females. That means that charges should be low, that opening hours should be compatible with the timetables of those most likely to seek help, and above all that there should be a friendly atmosphere and an assurance of confidentiality. To ensure that the services will meet the necessary criteria, it is important to ascertain the perceptions of the potential and actual clients, the attitudes of the health service providers, and the discrepancies between the two.

(i) *Contraception*

A careful assessment of needs, circumstances, and life-style is necessary in order to determine the best method in each case. The advantages and disadvantages of different methods have been widely discussed in the literature (*82, 83*). While, in many societies, there is considerable resistance to the provision of means of contraception to young people, in view of the increase in sexual activity among the young, the alternative may be unprotected intercourse with its attendant dangers of sexually transmitted diseases, unwanted pregnancy, induced abortion, and/or hazardous childbirth.

(ii) *Obstetrical services*

A pregnant adolescent should be seen as early in her pregnancy as possible to permit screening for risks such as hypertension or pelvic abnormality, to ensure adequate nutrition, and to enable changes to be monitored. Her attendance also provides an opportunity for counselling and for seeing that delivery takes place in the best conditions. In some instances, particularly if the mother is unmarried, it may be necessary to arrange for the baby to be adopted.

(iii) *Induced abortion*

Induced abortion is still a controversial matter in many societies, though by no means all. However, because sexual activity among the young is increasing, while contraception is often unavailable or inaccessible to them and no method is infallible, unwanted and dangerous pregnancies will occur. In these circumstances, there are many reasons why an adolescent may try to have her pregnancy terminated. Finding herself with an unexpected and unwanted pregnancy, she may face the prospect of having a child too early in life with a consequent disruption of educational and economic opportunities, psychosocial development, and chances of marriage. There is also the risk that pregnancy and delivery when she is not reproductively mature may damage her health. Circumstances may make it impossible to provide adequate care for a child born to a very young mother, and thus a cycle of poverty and ill-health could begin. Where a safe abortion is difficult to obtain because of legal restrictions, women throughout the world have resorted to illegal abortion in circumstances dangerous to health and to life itself. The risk is especially great for adolescents, who tend to seek abortion at a late stage of gestation. Counselling is vital to help reach the best decision within a given cultural context and to create circumstances that will prevent the recurrence of unwanted pregnancies.

(iv) *Sexually transmitted diseases*
The epidemic scale of the sexually transmitted diseases makes it urgent that accessible screening and treatment be widely provided, particularly in urban environments. Because of the stigma attached to these diseases, and because adolescents are most likely to be frightened and inexperienced in seeking treatment for them, a special effort must be made to ensure a confidential approach.

(v) *Services for men*
It has long been recognized that young men (whether as individuals or in the context of the couple) have been badly neglected in the provision of services in the area of reproductive health. This is mainly because of the obviously greater problems posed for women by pregnancy, but the sharing of responsibility by men for decisions in the area of reproductive health and for family planning in its broadest sense needs encouragement. Young people are often more responsive to new ideas and today's younger generation may be readier than its predecessors to share responsibility and decision-making more equitably within the couple.

6.2.2 *Nutrition*

Nutrition is an area in which young people can play an active and significant role. They can do so in the three following ways:

—*Participation in food production.*
By working on farms, young people obtain food for personal consumption, make money, learn new farming techniques and contribute to the community at large.
—*Participation in nutrition education.*
Information on food and nutrition may be acquired at school or in some community project. Young people may then take such information, e.g., what constitutes a well-balanced and nutritious meal, back to their families.
—*Participation in supplementary food programmes.*
Young people can contribute to the dissemination of information on nutrition or take part in the actual distribution of iron and vitamin supplements to people threatened with nutritional deficiency. Supplementation of the diet of teenage primigravidae with iron, folic acid, and antimalarials has been shown to result in better maternal and fetal growth (Harrison, K.A. et al., unpublished observations).

6.2.3 *Smoking*

In 1979, a WHO Expert Committee (*84*) stated that legislation to curb smoking would encroach upon the freedom of the individual less than any other conventional legislation relating to health measures. Legislation on smoking is, however, often strongly opposed by vested commercial interests. The measures relating to young people may be summed up as follows:

—prohibition of the sale of tobacco to minors;
—prohibition of smoking in places often frequented by children;
—restrictions on advertising;
—restrictions on cigarette sales from automatic vending machines.

But positive measures are needed as well. Entertainment and sports are particularly appropriate vehicles for incorporating health messages into young people's daily lives. Radio, television, and feature films that include scenes in which the leading characters refuse cigarettes (instead of the more common scenes where they smoke) would be a step in the right direction. An anti-smoking campaign in Scotland in 1982 included sponsorship of the national football team in the World Cup. The team had made a public statement emphasizing its non-smoking character, employing the slogan "The squad don't smoke". The Executive Board of WHO encouraged other teams to follow this example (*85*), and Czechoslovakia, Kuwait, New Zealand, and Northern Ireland responded positively. In addition, more innovative approaches, such as role-playing, could be adopted in anti-smoking programmes in schools.

6.2.4 *Alcohol abuse*

Given the many factors involved in alcohol consumption by young people, prevention and treatment are problematic. Better communication between field workers (especially health teams) and researchers and the abandonment of cross-sectional surveys in favour of longitudinal prospective studies of drinking patterns are recommended (*86*).

The identification of risk factors having predictive power is essential for prevention. However, as a wide variety of factors are involved and as drinking patterns vary considerably, the prevention, treatment, and alleviation of problems of alcohol abuse are difficult to institute. A well-planned strategy with appropriate coordination between the various relevant agencies is needed. Society must address the many ethical, legal, and regulatory issues involved in alcohol advertising and the availability of alcohol to the young. Families as well as professional health workers must be able to recognize incipient problems of alcohol dependence.

6.2.5 *Drug abuse*

Traditional methods of health education in which the dangers of drug use are pointed out may not be sufficient to prevent drug abuse. Preventive education may be most effective if it treats young people as individuals responsible for their own actions and encourages full discussion in a non-judgemental atmosphere. As with smoking, any publicity that makes drug use less fashionable will have an impact on the young.

For drug-dependent young people, training for employment has proved to be of enormous therapeutic and practical value by helping to ensure their successful re-entry into society (*87*).

6.2.6 *Rehabilitation of the disabled*

There are many possible approaches to the rehabilitation of disabled young people. Where there are professional health workers trained in rehabilitation techniques, modern technology, an adequate infrastructure, and sophisticated facilities for education and training, the options for rehabilitation are numerous. However, even where resources are limited, as in most developing countries, a variety of useful approaches, such as those listed below can be employed:

(*a*) ensuring that new buildings are accessible for the disabled from the outset;

(*b*) promoting the use of alternative technology and local materials to produce rehabilitation aids that are simpler and less costly;

(*c*) mobilizing family members and primary health care workers to assist in the delivery of medicaments, the use of simple physiotherapy, and the provision of intellectual and social stimuli;

(*d*) providing some form of gainful employment for disabled young people, preferably within the local community;

(*e*) mobilizing disabled adolescents themselves as promoters of preventive health measures, e.g., immunization against poliomyelitis or the provision of vitamin A supplements to prevent xerophthalmia;

(*f*) educating the general public about the needs of the disabled, especially the need for them to be treated as individuals.

6.2.7 *Health promotion at the place of work*

Certain health problems of young people can be avoided in the first place if there is appropriate job placement, i.e., a matching of the needs of the job with the abilities and potential of the individual. A pre-employment examination can also avert certain difficulties, for example, when prospective employees are allergic to various substances.

Young people should be protected, as far as possible, from dangerous working environments, e.g., areas where there is fast-moving machinery. Where there are toxic substances such as lead dust, the monitoring of the concentrations of these substances in the air, as well as in blood and urine, becomes important. Record-keeping can be used to indicate sickness and absence that might point to specific difficulties or low morale. Discrimination against women and minorities in employment should be eliminated.

Health promotion in the places of work should involve education about the broader issues of accident prevention, nutrition, family planning, and drug abuse. The early treatment and subsequent rehabilitation of young people with injury and illness, whether physical or psychological, should be ensured.

6.2.8 *Prevention of risks to future health*

Adolescence is a crucial time for preventive measures. Certain conditions or types of behaviour appearing during adolescence, though of minor importance at the time, may have serious consequences for health in later years. The early onset of obesity, hypertension, hyperlipidaemia, and diabetes mellitus, for example, are significant in this sense, as is the acquisition of habits in regard to the use of drugs and alcohol, sleep, and physical activity.

Adolescents are, to some extent, able to shape their own health patterns as well as those of the next generation. Adolescence provides a crucial access point for the improvement of health in adult life and in the next generation, an issue of great importance to society.

6.3 Young people and primary health care

A strategy for the enhancement of the health of young people and their communities that commands widespread support is that of primary health care carried out with the participation of the young. While their involvement can offer great benefits in the long-term, it cannot be initiated without considerable support from health agencies and other sectors, plus an empathetic response by health providers. Appropriate information, education, training, and support are necessary at the outset to ensure successful participation. The potential gains from this approach are considerable: a wider population coverage can be achieved than is possible at present, while young people can gain new skills, enhance their self-esteem, and use their energies constructively. By exercising responsibility and sharing in decisions about their own health care, they can help to make the services even more relevant. Primary health care must be backed up by secondary and tertiary levels of care as well, though a strong preventive programme will reduce pressure on the more expensive and specialized services provided at those levels.

6.4 Towards self-reliance in health care

Health issues relating to young people may be examined from several standpoints. Since the aim of this report is to provide guidance and to stimulate action in the context of primary health care, the Study Group proposed a classification of health issues based on the degree of individual and community self-reliance that may be achieved by endowing the community as far as possible with the relevant knowledge, skills, techniques, and authority.

To deal with any health issue in a community requires resources. At the least these must include information and some form of social support and reinforcement. Additional resources required include skills (biotechnical, communication, and clinical), materials such as drugs, expendable supplies, equipment, and physical facilities. With these requirements in mind, the Study Group proposed the following classification of the levels of care that might suitably be provided in a health programme:

- —self-care;
- —care provided by youth;
- —as above, but linked to health institutions;
- —institutionally supported health care, with youth participation.

In the less formal levels of care, where the emphasis is on prevention, information and social support are needed. More formalized care is likely to be curative in emphasis requiring more technical materials and skills, which render it more costly. The health sector must be able to provide technically sound information, monitor the provision of materials, and provide technical skills, facilities, and equipment, depending on the level of care.

Some examples of the types of health issue that might be dealt with at each level of care are listed below:

(a) *Self-care*
- —smoking
- —poor eating habits

(b) *Care provided by youth organizations*
- —alcohol abuse

—risk-taking behaviour leading to accidents or unwanted pregnancies

—weight disorders

—adjustment to stress reactions

(*c*) *Care provided by youth organizations with linkages to health institutions*

—occupational health problems

—pregnancy

—sexually transmitted disease

—suicidal behaviour

—post-accident disability

(*d*) *Institutionally supported health care, with youth participation*

—communication and speech disorders

—anomalies of growth and development

—abortion

—acute and chronic pelvic inflammatory disease

—sexually deviant behaviour

—depressive illness/schizophrenia

—chronic illness and disability.

The healthy development of young people can perhaps best be promoted through community-developed and community-based youth centres that employ a holistic approach to the needs of the young, rather than treat each need in isolation. Such an approach works best with young people and makes it possible to go beyond the individual's immediate problems to their causes and to facilitate his or her development.

The participation of young people in planning and providing services is an important factor. The young users of multiservice centres usually see themselves as members of a club where services are available, rather than as traditional clinic patients. Easy access, a flexible structure, a relaxed friendly atmosphere, and the opportunity to be involved in a variety of activities contribute to this impression. A high level of commitment, flexibility, and the ability to take risks are among the qualities required by those working in these centres.

The sensitization of health workers to the special needs of young people is particularly important. Their ability to listen to and respect the feelings of the young, to involve them in decision-making, to share information, and to transfer skills is essential to the success of the approach to health care just outlined, and training in the necessary techniques should be provided.

6.5 Some examples of youth participation

While there is growing recognition that it is both necessary and valuable for people to help provide their own health care, this new development needs strengthening. Below are some examples of the involvement of young people in the provision of care.

In Nigeria, under the National Youth Service Corps programme, initiated in 1973, all graduates of universities and other post-secondary institutions are required to serve the nation for one year after graduation. Their work during that year involves service in their own specialties in both rural and urban areas and participation in community development programmes, such as surveying needs and resources in the community and helping in building projects. Among other achievements, the programme has made it possible for rural areas to have doctors.

The Women's Centre Project for Adolescent Mothers in Jamaica (*88*) is an example of an innovative participatory approach to the health needs of young people in the broader context of their educational and employment needs. It was started by the Jamaican Women's Bureau to permit continuity of education for pregnant schoolgoers between the ages of 12 and 16 who, because of social censure, have been forced to withdraw from school. The programme strongly emphasizes practical education in family life and encourages active group discussion and participation. It also involves the putative fathers in an important programme designed to make young Jamaican men more aware of their role in the family and the responsibilities involved. Between 1978 and 1981, more than 400 young women took part in the project, and over two-thirds of them successfully returned to school. One of the major results of the project is the way in which it has strengthened the self-esteem of the participants, their capacity to plan, and their sense of having some control over the future. Not only has the Women's Centre had an impact on Jamaica, but it is serving as an example for other nations in the Caribbean area that are seeking to promote the health of adolescents.

In England, the Family Planning Association established "Grapevine" as an experimental project in two inner-city boroughs of London where the out-of-wedlock birth rate is twice the national average. It makes use of a communications network reaching out through other services, as well as word-of-mouth advertising, to bring help to those young people who typically tend to stay away from conventional services. Young people from 16 to 30 years of age take part in preventive health and sex education programmes, which are carried out among peer groups to ensure the relevance of the information. There are volunteer helpers, each specializing in a particular type of work, e.g., activities in pubs, youth clubs, or the street, or telephone work in the Centre itself. Volunteers also take part in the planning, and decision-making processes, in the induction of new volunteers, and in leading certain work groups. The professional staff work in liaison with statutory and voluntary agencies. The service is continually monitored to see what modifications may be needed and also to evaluate its appropriateness as a model for activities in other areas.

"The Door—A Centre of Alternatives", was established in New York, USA, in 1972 on the recommendation of a group of young professionals who felt that the vital needs of urban youth could be met only by a new approach to youth services. "The Door" was created as a model to demonstrate the effectiveness of comprehensive, integrated services and of networks or linkages between existing service systems. More than 400 young people from all over the New York metropolitan area come to "The Door" daily. There a wide range of activities and services are available to them. These are easily accessible and assembled under one roof in a setting architecturally designed to permit appropriate privacy in a friendly atmosphere. To thousands of disadvantaged adolescents, "The Door" has become a viable alternative to life-styles that are self-destructive, providing an acceptable source of help for young people who are unable or unlikely to approach the traditional agencies and institutions.

At "The Hub", a centre for teenagers in South Bronx, New York, USA, young people were hired to be trained in conducting interviews, gathering information, and assessing the needs of local youth. Drug abuse and teenage pregnancy emerged as the main problems facing young people in this troubled community. Young people helped plan a new youth health programme, which has now evolved into a peer education programme.

The Adolescent Orientation Centres (CORA) in Mexico City and neighbouring areas, which started in 1978, employ a multiservice approach to the needs of adolescents. Pilot preventive programmes offer promotional, educational, medical, psychological, cultural, and recreational activities to normal adolescents aged 11–19 years. Family planning services, sex information and counselling, and gynaecological services are also available. Through the family planning services, other services are offered in an attractive, "social club" atmosphere that is fun and healthy, rather than that of a traditional clinic. The activities of CORA include an outreach programme and the active involvement of young people in local community development.

In Canada, the Regina Multiservice Centre for Youth provides another example of youth participation. Since 1982, a developmental team made up of concerned community residents, specialists in problems of adolescence, and youth leaders have been engaged in planning an innovative, community-based, multiservice centre for young people in Regina. Young people are involved in the planning of the services designed for them and, to some extent, in the provision of these services. The staff include specially trained young people. Rather than being specifically problem-oriented, the centre focuses on facilitating normal growth and development. Through youth workers and leadership training programmes, young people who are ready to assume leadership roles among their peers are able to voice their opinions, to design and carry out projects, and to be of service to other young people and the community.

The High Risk Youth Project in Los Angeles, USA, combines the resources of the Children's Hospital of Los Angeles and Los Angeles Free Clinic to provide help for high-risk adolescents. The target population of runaways and street youngsters faces a variety of health and social problems. Workers from the indigenous services include adolescents who receive training prior to offering peer counselling.

One of the oldest established organizations involving young people is the World Association of Girl Guides and Girl Scouts (WAGGGS) which comprises 104 member organizations with a total membership of more than 8 million individual members. Essential features of their activities include: accepting personal responsibility for their health, self-discipline, and development; accepting various kinds of responsibility in their own communities (serving others, helping those handicapped by lack of education, or by ill health or financial difficulty); and the sharing of responsibility between men and women. The emphasis is on self-development and learning by doing volunteer work. Through their international network, the member organizations can help one another: for example, when the Girl Guides of Upper Volta (now Burkina Faso) ran out of funds for their well-digging project, they were assisted by the Girl Guides of Canada. The work done by the Association of Girl Guides in Zambia to change attitudes towards those suffering from Hansen's disease may also be cited. In similar ways, the Boy Scout organizations throughout the world encourage young people to join in helping others as part of their own self-development.

In May 1983, the First International Workshop on Comprehensive Youth Services and Youth Advocacy, held in Toronto, Canada, brought together young people, programme administrators, youth workers, and health workers from Australia, Canada, Chile, Colombia, Mexico, Panama, and the USA. The Conference, at which 22 programmes were represented, recognized the importance of a comprehensive approach to the development of youth services and the active involvement of young people in programme planning and service provision.

6.6 Guidelines for the active participation of young people in health service provision

While the activities described above differ widely in the particular needs they seek to meet and in the specific methods adopted, there is a strong common thread running through them all, namely the recognition that young people are a valuable resource in the promotion of health and well-being, both for others and for themselves. It is clear that, if this resource is to be used to the best advantage, young people must share responsibility for the relevant planning and decision-making. In this way, they will be motivated to help and the services they provide will have greater relevance for the other young people at whom they are aimed. There is great scope throughout the world for the wider utilization of this human resource. Whenever their cooperation has been sought, the young have responded enthusiastically and with measurable success. By appealing to the imagination of youth in fresh ways, it will surely be possible to evolve new and effective services.

Prerequisites for effective participation include: the selection of motivated youngsters, sound training, open communication, clearly presented information, a non-judgemental atmosphere, and the recognition that much can be learned from young people themselves. As a wide range of problems are likely to be presented, it would be

extremely useful to have the backing of an adult multidisciplinary
team, but the services themselves can often best be provided by
young people trained to help their peers on the basis of their own
experience.

It is important to ensure that:

(*a*) there are channels of communication permitting the full
access of the young people concerned to the information they need
in order to make decisions, and giving them an opportunity to feed
back their own ideas;

(*b*) the young people have an opportunity to strengthen their
organizational skills by participating in management;

(*c*) the young people have a *real* say in decisions affecting
objectives, policy, the nature of activities, and the allocation of
resources;

(*d*) they share in the responsibility for the economic, social, and
political consequences of their participation (*89*).

To achieve these goals, the professional workers who are inviting
the young people to join them in their activities should be sensitive
to their feelings and views and careful not to underestimate their
potential. If trusted, they will become more responsible, to
everyone's benefit.

6.7 Participation and life-style

The participation of young people in caring at various levels for
their own health and that of other members of the community
affirms the value of youth. It establishes adolescents and adults as
partners and provides a foundation for joint action, based on their
respective strengths and competence. Furthermore, it acknowledges
the teenager's "authority of experience" and the validity of
experiential learning as an aspect of self-help.

But the promotion of health by and among young people is
inextricably linked with their life-styles. An effective programme in
this area must be based on a clear understanding of the factors
determining the life-styles that manifest themselves at work, in
leisure, and in personal relationships. This holistic approach is
essential if life-styles that are detrimental to health are to be changed
(*90*).

Different health promotion strategies are required for different
situations. In structured environments, such as the school and the

work-place, there is scope for measures related to the activities carried out in these settings, for example, a modification of the school curriculum to include information relevant to adolescent life-styles, or the provision of specific safety information on the job. It is important that a system of social and psychological support should be available to back up these measures. In the less institutionalized social settings of the community, health promotion must concentrate on the participation and self-organization of young people according to their perceived needs and interests. In such circumstances, encouragement of the assessment of youth by youth is doubly advantageous, for not only is it likely to provide more reliable information, given adequate support, but it also engages young people themselves in self-help.

Programmes should be based on a positive concept of health that involves the capacity to communicate and express oneself, be creative, and change oneself and one's environment in a positive way. It also means dealing with the pains and problems of life in a constructive way instead of protecting oneself. The healthy young person is one who is able to realize his or her potential for personal growth and fulfilment and contribute to the community.

An approach limited to warnings about risk factors and specific models of behavioural change is inadequate for the promotion of healthier life-styles. Health promotion must rather develop comprehensive ways of supporting young people in dealing both with their individual developmental tasks and with the social issues relating to work, leisure, and peace that are of particular concern to them.

6.8 The role of the media in health promotion

Health information is essential for young people, but it will not get across if transmitted only through conventional channels. These channels are often dull and identified with the established authorities of the adult world, of whom the young are sometimes mistrustful and critical. In any case, they tend to be underutilized, as adolescents rarely seek information about health matters.

It is important to start health education before adolescence, as children will readily accept it as part of their schooling. It is equally important that adults should be informed of what adolescents want to know and what they perceive as their problems—subjects on which research is frequently needed.

In order to be listened to by adolescents, adults should use the language of young people and avoid communicating in a condescending manner. Young people need to have their own questions answered before being given information society thinks they need. The messages given by adults to the young must be clear and without ambiguity. It is essential that communication be two-way so that adolescents can express their own experience, as well as being the recipients of information adults wish to convey to them. Effective communication requires a non-judgemental atmosphere marked by mutual respect.

To inform young people, all methods are good, the old as well as the new, as long as nothing is forced on them. Information must be proposed, not imposed, through the greatest possible number of channels to which youth has easy access (a kind of self-service approach). Peers are often the best conveyors of health information, since young people will more readily listen to them.

Full use should be made of modern media, but not only the mass media. Provision must also be made for small-scale, inter-active programmes of communication. Where resources permit, video, audio, and photographic information on health should be provided in the framework of young people's social activities (at school, in youth clubs, churches, etc.); there should be full participation of the young people themselves and discussion should be encouraged.

Good vehicles for health promotion are music and drama, folk music and rock, the theatre, and video recordings. Popular music idols and sports heroes are often the ideal conveyors of health information to young people, who are particularly receptive to what they have to say.

6.9 Some research needs

The participation of young people in health promotion is a new area, in which it is necessary from the outset to explore innovations, monitor changes, and evaluate services through research. Both qualitative and quantitative research is appropriate. Modern research techniques based on a transdisciplinary approach will permit the use of small samples and qualitative measurements with scientific rigour.

In strengthening health services for young people, consideration must be given to the particular circumstances in deciding whether it is best to provide broad-based services or specialized ones, since each type has its own advantages. It may well be that the wider-ranging approach is best at the primary, less formal levels of health care, while specialization is more suitable to the secondary and tertiary levels. Research and evaluation should be carried out to ascertain the arrangements most suited to local needs, taking the views and experience of the young people themselves into account.

Another important question needing research is whether services should be exclusively health-oriented or be incorporated in youth centres already offering facilities for leisure pursuits, sports, training, or education. No doubt, either arrangement could be of value, but, again it is necessary to test the relative advantages and cost-effectiveness empirically. The possibility of going to a centre that does not automatically identify a young person as somebody with a health problem may make it easier for certain adolescents to overcome their anxieties. Other resources can be tapped with a view to modifying such centres to meet health needs.

There is a particular need for research on the best ways of incorporating the views of young people in the planning and implementation of health care. For this it will be necessary to utilize research designs that determine the interactions between the different parties to health care systems: the policy makers, the administrators and managers, the service providers, and the clients and potential clients (*80*). In some circumstances, young people may appropriately be represented in all four groups. The subjective perceptions of the interacting groups, the beliefs they hold about what is or ought to be provided, the degree to which their opinions coincide or disagree, and the nature of the disagreements are substantive data open to rigorous scientific exploration.

Finally, any research programme with the ultimate aim of promoting the health of the young must provide for liaison with those responsible for making and implementing decisions, if it is to have an impact. It should be viewed, not as a "one-off" project, but rather as an ongoing means of monitoring how far the goals of health promotion among the young are being met.

6.9.1 *Some questions for investigators*

—How far has your country formulated policies and strategies aimed at providing "Health for all by the year 2000"?

—In your country's policies on health services, what attention is given to the particular problems and needs of young people? Is there a youth policy?

—What emphasis is placed in your country on primary health care both by the general health services and by those more specifically concerned with young people?

—Within your country, region, or district, what data exist on young peoples' health and what data are needed to complete the picture?

—Is it possible to compile a profile on the young people in your area, indicating their physical growth and health, nutritional condition, housing, education, employment, etc.?

—Can you provide a comprehensive list of the health and health-related problems affecting young people in your area?

—How is information on young people currently collected in your country? What information gaps exist and how could they best be filled?

—Can you describe the ways in which health services are organized and monitored in your country, and how these services are relevant to the health and needs of young people?

—Is it possible to establish the characteristics of that percentage of young people in your country who utilize existing health services? Are these traditional or modern services? Are the characteristics of those young people who do not use any services different?

—How do your country's health and health-related services advertise their availability and range? Are there any programmes to inform young people of the services available?

—Are young people in your country actively involved in primary health care within their own communities? If there is no such involvement, how might it best be encouraged and developed?

—What kind of resources would be needed to support a health programme organized and predominantly staffed by young people, with the backing of health care workers and experts in the form of advice and guidance?

—Is there any training in your country for health care workers and other primary care workers to help them function more effectively with young people? If no such training exists, how might it best be organized?

—What research is there into health programmes for young people in your country, what provision is made for the evaluation of such programmes, and what are the needs in these areas?

7. CONCLUSIONS AND RECOMMENDATIONS

7.1 General policy considerations

Over the last decade, consultative groups convened by WHO have repeatedly recommended the development of national health policies to deal with issues affecting young people (*1*).[1] One of the themes of International Youth Year is participation. This is the new perspective from which the subject must be treated: the development of health care policy, *with* young people as active participants in the process, not merely the objects of it. It may be useful to consider the context in which this may take place.

Mention has been made of the relatively low position occupied by health in the concerns of today's young people, who tend to give priority to anxiety about lack of training and educational opportunities, unemployment, the future of humankind, the search for a role in shaping personal and societal destiny, and questions of equity and justice. This should not, however, deter efforts to enlist the participation of the young in matters of health policy for it is only through sound health that the other issues can be fully dealt with.

This, then, is the proper backdrop against which to consider the subject. The challenge is that of empowering young people to become active participants in policy development and promoting them as advocates of health care policies appropriate to their own needs and perceptions—in fact, enabling them to become an active force, or constituency, for change.

Health policy has historically been made by an elite that was often remote from the groups most affected. The pattern has been for adult providers of health care to formulate the issues as they perceive them from various disciplinary angles, and to deal with them accordingly. What is being proposed is that today's advocates of a

---

[1] *Regional working group on health needs of adolescents: final report*. Manila, WHO Regional Office for the Western Pacific, 1980 (unpublished document, ICP/MCH/005).

health care policy geared to youth should join hands with young people in promoting change.

In the course of its deliberations, the Study Group singled out a number of areas within the broad range of topics covered to form the basis of its recommendations. Some of the recommendations are new, and some reinforce the consensus of previous meetings.

What emerged very strongly was the conviction that attitudes must change so that young people come to be considered as a resource rather than a problem. In addition, it was unanimously agreed that, given the appropriate and necessary support and encouragement, young people can deal with many of their own health problems and, at the same time, contribute significantly to the health and well-being of the community at large.

7.2 General recommendations

The Study Group recommended:

(*a*) that priority be given at the international, national, and local levels to making those who influence the health of the young more sensitive both to their special needs and to their special qualities;

(*b*) that young people participate and share in the responsibility for developing policies and planning strategies for the promotion of their own health;[1]

(*c*) that young people be trained for, and actively involved in, the implementation of such policies through the provision of services, information, education, and counselling to people of their own age, and other segments of the community in need;

(*d*) that young people be given the opportunity to strengthen the positive aspects of their life-styles and be helped to prepare for their future responsibilities as marital partners and as parents;

(*e*) that, in promoting the health of the young, an intersectoral approach be adopted, since only then can the social, economic, political, and cultural conditions in which young people live be taken into account;

(*f*) that further support be given to the programmes that already focus on the needs of young people, e.g., those dealing with the problems associated with smoking, alcohol and drug abuse, sexual and reproductive health, and abnormal risk-taking;

---

[1] An earlier WHO meeting actually involved young people: see May et al. (*91*).

(*g*) that, in view of the current paucity of the data necessary for planning and implementing health services relevant to the young, procedures be developed for collecting and disseminating such data;

(*h*) that research be conducted to establish norms of health development for young people and identify their special needs and problems, that young people themselves actively participate in such research, and that comparisons be made of adolescents and young people who have successfully adapted to change, as well as of those with difficulties, within and across cultures;

(*i*) that sound knowledge about, and respect for, the capabilities of youth be promoted by popular methods using the full range of media and other techniques;

(*j*) that full use be made of International Youth Year to promote the concept of youth outlined in this report, since it is essential to the achievement of Health for All by the Year 2000.

7.3 Recommendations for specific action

The Study Group recommended:

(*a*) that an international clearing-house on young people's health be established to provide sound information on norms, special problems, and programmes of participation by young people in the promotion of health and well-being, special material aimed at the young, the names of people and institutions responsible for questions of young people's health and the coordination of activities in this area in governmental and non-governmental agencies;

(*b*) that curricula and training programmes be developed for professional workers in all sectors dealing with young people and their special needs, in areas such as general development, sexuality and human reproduction, and risk-taking behaviour;

(*c*) that innovations involving young people's participation in the delivery of health care, particularly at the primary level, be explored in order to improve health promotion in the family and community and, at the same time, reduce costs in the provision of services by preventing future problems;

(*d*) that an intersectoral approach be used to promote the health and wellbeing of young people at work and at play, through sports and youth clubs, volunteer programmes, and education and training, so that activities are coordinated, complementary, and cost-effective;

(*e*) that there should be sound and comprehensive educational programmes to facilitate the development of young people, to reduce unnecessary stress among them, to provide them with an appropriate understanding of sexual matters, including human reproduction and relationships, and to encourage them to adopt healthy life-styles;

(*f*) that, at the societal level, in policy-making, in legislation on education, health, social welfare, advertising, and other matters affecting young people, and especially in the use of the media, people should be made aware of the need to encourage the young in their particular strengths and reduce the pressures that lead to unhealthy life-styles.

7.4 Special recommendations on research

The Study Group recommended:

(*a*) that, in research on health services, their evaluation, and the introduction of modifications and innovations, care must be taken to ensure that the perceptions of young people and their assessment of the adequacy of the services in meeting their needs are taken into account;

(*b*) that baseline data be collected, wherever needed, on the norms of development appropriate to a particular society, including the biological and psychosocial aspects of maturation, and that national statistics about young people be made available for more finely graded age-specific groups;

(*c*) that a wide variety of techniques, including self-assessment and qualitative as well as quantitative measurements, where appropriate, be used to examine the special problems of young people;

(*d*) that research be encouraged into: the special problems of contemporary youth, including the effects of sexual activity on the psychosocially immature, the effects of migration from rural to urban areas, the effects of the pressure generated by the mass media, and the isolation of young people from their families as a result of industrialization; the interaction of nutrition and energy expenditure on menarche; the neuro-endocrine basis of mood changes in the young; the cross-cultural epidemiology of psychiatric disorders; and the situation of special groups at risk, including the unemployed, the socially disadvantaged, and the handicapped;

(*e*) that cross-cultural comparisons be made with a view to paving the way for a wider exchange of pertinent information on young people throughout the world, and that models of successful adaptation by young people, whether in less developed, transitional, or developed societies, be made available to all as potential models for the promotion of health;

(*f*) that the dissemination of the relevant research findings be promoted through all sectors of society by the best means possible, so that the product of sound research can be put to work for the benefit of all.

ACKNOWLEDGEMENTS

The Study Group gratefully acknowledges the special contributions to their work of: Dr L. Edouard, Consultant, Maternal and Child Health, WHO, Geneva, Switzerland; Mrs M. Romer, Maternal and Child Health, WHO, Geneva, Switzerland; and Dr N. Suarez-Ojeada, Regional Adviser in Maternal and Child Health and Family Planning, WHO Regional Office for the Americas, Washington, DC, USA. It also wishes to thank the following staff members of WHO, Geneva, Switzerland, for representing their respective divisions or units: Dr G.M. Antal, Bacterial and Venereal Infections; Dr D.E. Barmes, Noncommunicable Diseases; Ms P.M. Elmiger, Coordination; Ms R. Landy, Public Information and Education for Health; Dr J. Lau Hansen, Health Legislation; Dr A. Monoharan, Occupational Health; Dr C. Montoya-Aguilar, Strengthening of Health Services; Dr J. Orley, Mental Health; Mrs J. Peters, Health Education; Dr A. Pradilla, Nutrition; and Dr F. Siem Tjam, Strengthening of Health Services. The Study Group wishes to thank Dr P. Eisen, Richmond, Victoria, Australia, for preparing some of the background material. Special thanks are due to Dr Herbert L. Friedman, Consultant, Maternal and Child Health, WHO, Geneva, for his work in preparing this report for publication with the assistance of Ms Jane Ferguson.

REFERENCES

1. WHO Technical Report Series No. 583, 1975 (*Pregnancy and abortion in adolescence:* report of a WHO Meeting).
2. TANNER, J.M. Physical growth. In: Mussen, P.H., ed. *Carmichael's manual of child psychology,* 3rd ed., New York, Wiley, 1970, vol 1, pp. 77–155.
3. SIZONENKO, P.C. Endocrinology in preadolescents and adolescents. I. Hormonal changes during normal puberty. *American journal of diseases in childhood,* **132**: 704–712 (1978).
4. HIRSCH, M. ET AL. Emission of spermatozoa, age of onset. *International journal of andrology,* **2**: 289 (1979).
5. WORLD HEALTH ORGANIZATION. A multicentre cross-sectional study of menarche. *Journal of adolescent health care* (in press).

6. FRISCH, R. & REVELLLE, R. Height and weight at menarche and a hypothesis of menarche. *Archives of disease in childhood,* **49**: 695–701 (1971).

7. BILLEWICZ, W.Z. ET AL. Comments on the critical metabolic mass and age of menarche. *Annals of human biology,* **3**: 51–59 (1976).

8. MONEY, S. & EHRHARDT, A.A. *Men and women: boy and girl. The differentiation and dimorphism of gender identity from conception to maturity.* Baltimore, John Hopkins University Press, 1972.

9. RUTTER, M. Psychosexual development. In: Rutter, M., ed. *Scientific foundations of developmental psychiatry.* London, Heinemann, 1979, pp. 322–339.

10. PIAGET, J. Piaget's theory. In: Mussen, P.H., ed. *Carmichael's manual of child psychology.* 3rd ed., New York, Wiley, 1970, vol. 1, pp. 703–732.

11. RUTTER, M. ET AL. Adolescent turmoil: fact or fiction. *Journal of child psychology and psychiatry,* **17**: 35–56 (1976).

12. SOMMER, B.B. *Puberty and adolescence.* Oxford, Oxford University Press, 1978.

13. KEYFITZ, N. The impact of modernization. In Lengyel, P. ed., *Approaches to the science of socioeconomic development.* Paris, United Nations Educational, Scientific, and Cultural Organization, 1971, pp. 89–98.

14. BANKS, J.A. *Prosperity and parenthood.* London, Routledge and Kegan Paul, 1954.

15. LENGYEL, P., ed. *Approaches to the science of socioeconomic development.* Paris, United Nations Educational, Scientific, and Cultural Organization, 1971.

16. EISENSTADT, S.N., ed. *Comparative perspectives on social change.* Boston, Little, Brown, 1968.

17. BRENNER, M.H. *Mental illness and the economy.* Cambridge, MA, Harvard University Press, 1973.

18. HARRIS, R.D. Unemployment and its effect on the teen-ager. *Australian family physician,* **9**: 546–553 (1980).

19. HENDERSON, S. ET AL. *Neurosis and the social environment.* Sydney, Academic Press, 1981.

20. REES, W. Medical aspects of unemployment. *British medical journal,* **283**: 1630–1631 (1981).

21. RUTTER, M. *Changing youth in a changing society.* London, Nuffield Provincial Hospitals Trust, 1979.

22. GOODE, W.J. Industrialization and family change. In: Eisenstadt, S.N., ed., *Comparative perspectives on social change.* Boston, Little, Brown and Co. 1968.

23. LEETE, R. New directions in family life. *Population trends,* **15**: 4–9 (1979).

24. WORLD HEALTH ORGANIZATION. *Basic documents,* 34th ed. Geneva, WHO, 1984.

25. DELIEGE, A. Indicators of physical, mental and social wellbeing. *World health statistics quarterly,* **36**: 349–393 (1983).

26. MAHLER, H. The meaning of "health for all by the year 2000". *World health forum,* **2**: 16 (1981).

27. MANOHARAN, A. A philosophy of health. *Centerview,* March 1982: 14–16 (1982).

28. BRUNSWICK, A.F. & JOSEPHSON, E. Adolescent health in Harlem. *American journal of public health,* Suppl., October 1972.

29. MICHAUD, P.A. & MARTIN, J. La santé des adolescents vaudois de 16 à 19 ans: leur perceptions, leur pratiques et leur souhaits. *Revue suisse de médecine (Praxis),* **49**: 1545–1553 (1983).

30. PARCEL, G.S. ET AL. Adolescent health concerns, problems and patterns of utilization in a triethnic urban population. *Pediatrics,* **60**: 157–164 (1977).

114

31. SCHONBERG, S.K. & COHEN, M.I. Health needs of the adolescent. Proceedings of the First International Symposium of the International College of Pediatrics, June 18–22, 1978. *Paediatrician,* **1** (suppl.): 131–140 (1979).

32. WHO Technical Report Series, No. 609, 1977 (*Health needs of adolescents:* report of a WHO Expert Committee).

33. JESSOR, R. & JESSOR, S.L. *Problem behaviour and psychological development.* New York, Academic Press, 1977.

34. PROJECTGRUPPE JUGENDBÜRO. *Die Lebenswelt von Hauptschülern.* München, Juventa, 1977.

35. ERBEN, L. ET AL. *Prevention, education and health beliefs. Sociological considerations on health education and health promotion, 1983* Background paper for the Tenth European Public Parliamentary Hearing on Health Economics, Council of Europe, Paris, 25–26 October 1983.

36. WHO Technical Report Series, No. 562, 1975 (*Services for cardiovascular emergencies:* report of a WHO Expert Committee), p. 7.

37. ADAMS, L. ET AL. Respiratory impairment induced by smoking in children in secondary schools, *British medical journal,* **288**: 891–895 (1984).

38. HAMMOND, E.C. Smoking in relation to the death rates of one million men and women. In: Haenszel, W., ed. *Epidemiological approaches to the study of cancer and other chronic diseases.* Bethesda, MD, National Cancer Institute, 1966 (National Cancer Institute Monograph 19).

39. TAHA, A. & BALL, K. Smoking in Africa: the coming epidemic. *World smoking and health,* **7**: 25–30 (1982).

40. UNITED STATES OF AMERICA. SURGEON GENERAL. *Smoking and health.* Washington, DC, United States Department of Health, Education and Welfare, 1979, pp. 17–14.

41. MOSER, J. Alcohol problems in children and adolescents: A growing threat. In: Jeanneret, O., ed. *Alcohol and youth,* Basel, Karger, 1983, p. 149.

42. DAVIES, J.B. Children's and adolescents' attitudes towards alcohol and alcohol-dependence. In: Jeanneret, O., ed. *Alcohol and youth,* Basel, Karger, 1983, pp. 42–53.

43. MOSER, J. *Prevention of alcohol-related problems: an international review of preventive measures, policies and programmes.* Toronto, Alcoholism and Drug Addiction Research Foundation, on behalf of WHO, 1980, p. 310.

44. MOSER, J. *Problems and programmes related to alcohol and drug dependence in 33 countries,* Geneva, 1974 (WHO Offset Publication No. 6).

45. DEVATHASON, G. ET AL. Complications of chronic glue (toluene) abuse in adolescents. *Australian and New Zealand journal of medicine,* **14**: 39–43 (1984).

46. VEERAGHAUAN, V. Drug use among university students. In: Mohan, D. et al., ed. *Current research on drug abuse in India.* Delhi, Mohan and Sethi, 1981, pp. 89–98.

47. HALPERIN, S.F. ET AL. Unintended injuries among adolescents and young adults: a review and analysis. *Journal of adolescent health care,* **4**: 275–281 (1983).

48. MANCIAUX, M. & JEANNERET, O. Accidents in childhood and adolescence: epidemiological approach and preventive measures. *Revue d'épidémiologie et de santé publique,* **31**: 433–444 (1983).

49. RABKIN, J. & STRUENING, E. Life events, stress and illness. *Science,* **194**: 1013–1020 (1976).

50. LAZARUS, R. & COHEN, J. Environmental stress. In: Altman, I. & Wohlwill, J., ed., *Human behaviour and environment.* New York, Plenum, 1977, vol. 2.

51. CASSEL, J. The contribution of the social environment to host residence. *American journal of epidemiology,* **109**: 107–123 (1976).
52. Adapted from a policy statement on health services for adolescents by the Department of Health, New South Wales, quoted in: Bennett, D.L. *Adolescent health in Australia, an overview of needs and approaches to care.* Glebe, Australian Medical Association, 1984.
53. HOLINGER, P.C. Adolescent suicide: an epidemiological study of recent trends. *American journal of psychiatry,* **135**: 754–756 (1978).
54. SAINSBURY, P. & JENKINS, J.S. The accuracy of officially reported suicide statistics for purposes of epidemiological research. *Journal of epidemiology and community health,* **36**: 43–48 (1982).
55. LADAME, F. & JEANNERET, O. Suicide in adolescence: some comments on epidemiology and prevention. *Journal of adolescence,* **5**: 355–366 (1982).
56. McCORMICK, M.L. ET AL. High-risk young mothers: infant mortality and morbidity in four areas in the United States, 1973–1978. *American journal of public health,* **74**: 18–23 (1983).
57. ROTHENBERG, P.B. & VARGA, P.E. The relationship between age of mother and child health and development. *American journal of public health,* **78**: 810–817 (1981).
58. McCORMICK, M.C. ET AL. Rehospitalization in the first year of life for high-risk survivors. *Pediatrics,* **66**: 991–999 (1980).
59. McCORMICK, M.C. ET AL. Injury and its correlates among 1 year old children. *American journal of disturbed children,* **135**: 159–163 (1981).
60. HARRISON, K.A. & ROSSITER, C.E. Zaria (Nigeria) maternal survey 1976–79 (supplement). *British journal of obstetrics and gynaecology* (in press).
61. SCHEDTER, M.D. & ROBERGE, L. Sexual exploitation. In: Helfer, R.E. & Kempe, C.H., ed. *Child abuse and neglect* Philadelphia, Baldinger Publishing Co., 1976, pp. 127–142.
62. KNORR, D. & BIDLINGMAIER, F. Gynecomastia in male adolescents. *Clinical endocrinology and metabolism,* **4**: 157 (1975).
63. SOUTHARM, A.L. & RICHART, R.M. The prognosis for adolescents with menstrual abnormalities. *American journal of obstetrics and gynecology,* **94**: 637–645 (1966).
64. HEALD, F.P. Nutrition in adolescence. In: Wallace, H.M. et al., ed. *Maternal and child health practices, problems, resources and methods of delivery.* Springfield, Charles & Thomas, 1973, pp. 838–850.
65. JEANNERET, O. & RAYMOMD, L. Habitudes alimentaires des adolescents—implications pour la prévention. *Revue suisse de médecine (Praxis),* **25**: 1137–1147 (1981).
66. BENGOA, J.M. Recent trends in the public health aspects of protein calorie malnutrition. *WHO Chronicle,* **24**: 609 (1970).
67. NAIDU, U. & PARASURAMAN, S. *Health situation of youth in India.* Bombay, Tata Institute of Social Sciences, 1982.
68. SUSKIND, R.M. Immune status in the malnourished host. *Journal of tropical pediatrics,* **26**: 1–6 (1980).
69. RICKARBY, G.A. Psychosocial dynamics in obesity. *Medical journal of Australia,* **2**: 602–605 (1981).
70. THURSTON, J.H. ET AL. Prognosis in childhood epilepsy, *New England journal of medicine,* **14**: 831–836 (1982).
71. ROBERTSON, S.I. ET AL. The implications of family dynamics in the management of the diabetic adolescent. In: Laron, Z. & Galatzer, A. *Psychological aspects of*

diabetes in children and adolescents. Pediatric and adolescent endocrinology, Basel, Karger, 1982, Vol. 10, pp. 83–88.

72. WRIGHT, B. *Physical disability—psychological approach*. New York, Harper, 1960.

73. INTERNATIONAL LABOUR OFFICE; *Report of the Director-General. International Labour Conference, 1983*, Geneva, ILO.

74. FORSSMAN, S. & COPEE, G.H. *Occupational health problems of young workers*. Geneva, International Labour Office, 1973 (Occupational Safety and Health Series, No. 26).

75. WORLD HEALTH ORGANIZATION. Hospitalization of mental patients. A survey of existing legislation. *International digest of health legislation*, **6**: 1–100 (1955).

76. CURRAN, W.J. & HARDING, T.W. The law and mental health: harmonizing objectives. *International digest of health legislation*, **28**: 725–886 (1977).

77. TIETZE, C. *Induced abortion: a world view, 1983*, 5th ed. New York, The Population Council, 1983, pp. 43–45.

78. COOK, R.J. & DICKENS, B.M. *Emerging issues in commonwealth abortion laws*. London, Commonwealth Secretariat, 1983, pp. 16–17.

78a. ROYSTON, E. & FERGUSON, J. The coverage of maternity care: a critical review of available information. *World health statistics quarterly*, **38**: 267–288 (1985).

79. WHO REGIONAL OFFICE FOR EUROPE. *Psychosocial factors related to accidents in childhood and adolescence. Report on a WHO Technical Group*, 1981 (EURO Reports and Studies No. 46), p. 6.

80. FRIEDMAN, H.L. & EDSTRÖM, K.G. *Adolescent reproductive health: an approach to health service research*. Geneva, World Health Organization, 1983 (WHO Offset Publication No. 77).

81. MCKAY, J. ET AL. *Adolescent fertility. Report of an international consultation*. London, International Planned Parenthood Federation, 1983.

82. BENNETT, D.L. *Adolescent health in Australia—an overview of needs and approaches to care*. Australian Medical Association, 1984.

83. FRASER, I.S. A perspective of the beneficial and adverse effects of oral contraceptives. *Current therapeutics* (in press).

84. WHO Technical Report Series, No. 636, 1979 (*Controlling the smoking epidemic*. Report of the WHO Expert Committee on Smoking Control).

85. WORLD HEALTH ORGANIZATION. *Handbook of resolutions and decisions of the World Health Assembly and the Executive Board. Volume II. 1973–1984*. Geneva, 1985, pp. 175–176 (EB69.R18).

86. JEANNERET, O. Drinking problems in adolescence: three issues in future field research. In: Jeanneret, O., ed. *Child health and development*, vol. 2. Basel, Karger, pp. 160–167, 1983.

87. SACKSTEIN, E. Drugs and youth: an international perspective on vocational and social reintegration. *United Nations bulletin on narcotics*, **33**: 34–35 (1980).

88. MCNEIL, P. ET AL. The Women's Centre in Jamaica: an innovative project for adolescent mothers. *Studies in family planning*, **14**: 143–149 (1983).

89. SHONE, J. & MCDERMOTT, J. *Youth 2009—local youth policy development process*. Youth Affairs Council of Victoria, Australia, 1980.

90. WORLD HEALTH ORGANIZATION. Health promotion and lifestyles: perspectives of the WHO Regional Office in Europe. *Hygie*, **1**: 57–60 (1982).

91. MAY, A.R. ET AL. *Mental health of adolescents and young persons. Report on a technical conference*. Geneva, World Health Organization, 1971 (Public Health Papers, No. 41).